THE
EVERYTHING®
PALEOLITHIC DIET
BOOK

Dear Reader,

The Everything® Paleolithic Diet Book is a book that represents years of searching for a level of health and well-being that transcends modern day fad diets. It took us a while to realize that there was no quick fix or magic fountain. Becoming healthy and fit was simply a matter of trusting the wisdom that our ancient ancestors possessed and a commitment to attaining that level of wellness.

This plan is not a diet and this book is not a diet plan. It is a guide to a lifestyle that brings your body back in sync with your genetics. Through the years, nothing has made us feel healthier, stronger, and more in balance with our inner selves. We feel and look better than ever, and it's all because of the Paleolithic journey. We are thrilled to share the years of knowledge we have culminated with you. We hope that after reading this book, you start your path to the healthiest YOU there is. It is possible. We are living proof!

In health,

Jodie Cohen

Gilaad Cohen

Welcome to the EVERYTHING® Series!

These handy, accessible books give you all you need to tackle a difficult project, gain a new hobby, comprehend a fascinating topic, prepare for an exam, or even brush up on something you learned back in school but have since forgotten.

You can choose to read an *Everything*® book from cover to cover or just pick out the information you want from our four useful boxes: e-questions, e-facts, e-alerts, and e-ssentials.

We give you everything you need to know on the subject, but throw in a lot of fun stuff along the way, too.

We now have more than 400 *Everything*® books in print, spanning such wide-ranging categories as weddings, pregnancy, cooking, music instruction, foreign language, crafts, pets, New Age, and so much more. When you're done reading them all, you can finally say you know *Everything*®!

QUESTION

Answers to common questions

FACT

Important snippets of information

ALERT

Urgent warnings

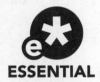

ESSENTIAL

Quick handy tips

PUBLISHER Karen Cooper

DIRECTOR OF ACQUISITIONS AND INNOVATION Paula Munier

MANAGING EDITOR, EVERYTHING® SERIES Lisa Laing

COPY CHIEF Casey Ebert

ASSISTANT PRODUCTION EDITOR Jacob Erickson

ACQUISITIONS EDITOR Lisa Laing

SENIOR DEVELOPMENT EDITOR Brett Palana-Shanahan

EDITORIAL ASSISTANT Ross Weisman

EVERYTHING® SERIES COVER DESIGNER Erin Alexander

LAYOUT DESIGNERS Colleen Cunningham, Elisabeth Lariviere, Ashley Vierra, Denise Wallace

THE
EVERYTHING®
PALEOLITHIC
DIET BOOK

An all-natural, easy-to-follow plan to:

- Improve health • Lose weight
- Increase endurance • Prevent disease

Jodie Cohen and Gilaad Cohen
Certified CrossFit Trainers and Coaches

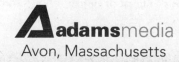
Avon, Massachusetts

This book is dedicated to our children,
Charlie and Olivia, who remind us daily
that living a healthy lifestyle is the greatest gift
to ourselves and to our family.

An Everything® Series Book.
Everything® and everything.com® are registered trademarks of F+W Media, Inc.

Published by Adams Media, a division of F+W Media, Inc.
57 Littlefield Street, Avon, MA 02322 U.S.A.
www.adamsmedia.com

ISBN 10: 1-4405-1206-X
ISBN 13: 978-1-4405-1206-3
eISBN 10: 1-4405-1268-X
eISBN 13: 978-1-4405-1268-1

Printed in the United States of America.

10 9 8 7 6 5 4 3 2 1

Library of Congress Cataloging-in-Publication Data
is available from the publisher.

The information in this book should not be used for diagnosing or treating any health problem. Not all diet and exercise plans suit everyone. You should always consult a trained medical professional before starting a diet, taking any form of medication, or embarking on any fitness or weight-training program. The author and publisher disclaim any liability arising directly or indirectly from the use of this book.

This publication is designed to provide accurate and authoritative information with regard to the subject matter covered. It is sold with the understanding that the publisher is not engaged in rendering legal, accounting, or other professional advice. If legal advice or other expert assistance is required, the services of a competent professional person should be sought.
—From a *Declaration of Principles* jointly adopted by a Committee of the American Bar Association and a Committee of Publishers and Associations

This book is available at quantity discounts for bulk purchases.
For information, please call 1-800-289-0963.

Contents

Acknowledgments

It is very difficult to get years of passion and research onto the printed page. I have lived this lifestyle so long that it's old hat for me. I didn't think about how difficult it could be to write it all down. If it weren't for the loved ones around me, this book would never have been completed.

First, I would like to thank my friend, Sher, who assured me that I had enough wonderful information to share with the world and that the world would have the desire to listen to what I had to say.

Many friends contributed to the wealth of recipes in this book. Shu-yee spent many days and nights in the kitchen slaving over Paleolithic recipes and experimenting with bold flavors to spice up dishes. Mackenzie, Danielle, Amy, Laura, Cristina, Grayson, Jenny, Michelle, Susie, and Adela added to the mix of fun and interesting recipes.

I wish to humbly thank the members of CrossFit Newton, who trust me with their Paleo journeys on a daily basis and give me the inspiration to continue learning and teaching about the Paleolithic lifestyle.

Without the wisdom of my dear friend and colleague, Jodi Jones of Modelper4mance.com, the bridge between nutrition and athletic performance would not have been built.

Finally, if I did not have Gil, my husband, by my side providing continuous love and support, this endeavor could not have been completed. I love you!

—JC

First I would like to thank all the athletes at CrossFit Newton for always inspiring me to better myself.

I would also like to thank my wife for being so dedicated to fitness, that I have no choice but to keep up with her.

Lastly, I wouldn't be where I am today if it weren't for the love and support of my friends and family.

—GC

Introduction

THE PALEOLITHIC LIFESTYLE IS not like most modern-day diet plans. In fact, it is probably the oldest diet in the world. This plan takes you back to the wisdom our ancient ancestors possessed before fast food, fast crops, and quick-fix diet pills existed. Back when hunting and gathering for food was the basis for survival. These hunter-gatherers were free of diabetes, obesity, heart disease, gastrointestinal disorders, and cancer. Their bodies were not inflamed and sick. They were lean, fit prehistoric athletes.

The health and diet industry has been flawed for quite some time. When something is wrong, medicines are given. When medication doesn't work, more medication is prescribed. Very few will take a deep look inside at the root of the problem. Treating the symptoms is faster and more profitable for the pharmaceutical companies and health industry. But, the symptoms linger, silent inflammation continues, and pains cease to subside.

The Paleolithic lifestyle gives you the tools you need to lose weight, gain muscle, and achieve peak athletic performance and optimum health. Your search for the one plan that will finally give you the answers you seek will finally end. This plan does it all. It will work for anyone with any issue. It will bring your body back in balance and make you feel like you did when you were young, full of life with boundless energy.

Human food choices have been evolving since the domestication of animals. As the world started to do things faster, quicker, and in greater numbers, quantity, not quality, became the primary focus. Sure, you can feed more people on a farm that uses poisons to kill pests and hormones to fatten up livestock, but are these additives healthy in our bodies? Are these harsh chemicals building up in our family's insides and making them sick? If you look at the rates of disease, cancer, diabetes, and obesity in the world, we really need to ask ourselves what is going wrong. Today's post agricultural world may feed more people, but it surely isn't giving them wholesome, nutrient dense options that help them have hearty immune systems to fend off sickness.

If you have wanted to increase your athletic performance, the Paleolithic plan has been shown to reduce overall body fat, decrease race times, and increase overall output. In the CrossFit community alone, athletes have been combining this diet regime with their training and seen unimaginable gains in strength, power, stamina, and many other fitness skills.

This lifestyle is gaining worthy popularity in the entire fitness community. In addition to athletic gains, overall health has improved, sickness rates have gone down, and quality of life has improved dramatically. Every athlete knows that at the base of all activity, nutrition is the foundation that keeps everything together. If this foundation is not solid, optimum performance will never be achieved. The Paleolithic lifestyle will give you the foundation needed to build your athletic potential. You will see gains that you would never have considered possible before, just from eating good, clean, organic foods. It really is that easy.

The Everything® Paleolithic Diet Book contains instructions to help you transfer to a healthier lifestyle. The extensive meal plans, shopping lists, and recipes will help to get you started on your way. You will learn how to eat as our primal ancestors did over 10,000 years ago without hunting down your next meal or picking fruits and vegetables from the garden daily. All you will need is a goal for a healthier lifestyle and a plan to set you on your way. It's that easy. The rewards are endless. Give yourself and your family the gift of optimal health. There is no gift worth more.

CHAPTER 1

An Introduction to the Paleolithic Lifestyle

The Paleolithic lifestyle is not a diet plan. It's not a fancy get-thin-quick scheme. It is simply a nutritional lifestyle that can make you healthier than you have ever been before. The Paleolithic lifestyle is a plan that can help you control body weight, lower body fat, reduce cholesterol, relieve gastrointestinal disorders and discomforts, combat diabetes, and fight cancer. If you have longed for a healthier and simpler alternative to current diets, this lifestyle is for you.

The Paleolithic Era

Who would have thought that eating like a caveman would be a good idea? Little did we know how much knowledge our Paleolithic ancestors possessed. Even though they had to find, hunt, and kill most of their food, they were still eating better than most of the world today. And, the exercise they received while hunting their food was the icing on the cake. The Paleolithic humans had it right, while people today are doing it all wrong. Today's diets are wreaking havoc on the human body.

Before the Neolithic time period where development of agriculture and the domestication of animals was commonplace, Paleolithic humans were forced to survive off the land. They hunted wild game for protein and gathered fruits, vegetables, nuts, and seeds. There were no grains harvested, legumes cooked, or milk past weaning. These people ate what they could find and they spent their lives hunting and gathering it. As a result they were free from the diet-based problems that current day diets are plagued by.

FACT

Modern day humans are only one tenth of 1 percent genetically different from our Paleolithic ancestors. During the last 10,000 years our diets have changed dramatically, yet humans have changed very little.

Hunter-Gatherers

There are still some hunter-gatherers in existence today. They are peoples sustaining themselves and their families off of the land just as our ancestors of the Pleistocene epoch. Today, some examples of traditional hunter-gatherers that continue this lifestyle are the Bushmen of southern Africa, the Pygmies of central Africa, and the Spinifex people of western Australia. These tribes are practically free of the common ailments and killers of our generation today: heart disease, diabetes, arthritis, and cancer. Once farming began, issues with tooth decay, shorter life spans, infant mortality, and iron deficiencies are recorded. These are not issues that hunter-gatherers frequently faced.

Why is it that today's hunter-gatherer tribes are healthier than the rest of the world? Their lives appear on the outside to be much more difficult. They do not have modern medicine, modern shelter, or modern conveniences. They have no refrigeration to keep food for long periods of time. Yet, they survive and live healthier lives than most of the world. Their genetic makeup is not different than the rest of the humans on earth. They are not a "super species" of humans. The secret is in their diet.

Today's Paleolithic Diet

So you're thinking that you need to move to the forest and take up hunting, fishing, and gardening to be on today's Paleolithic diet? That could not be further from the truth. The Paleolithic lifestyle simply requires a shift in your thinking. First, you will need to learn what foods are considered Paleo "yes" or Paleo "no." From there a simple shopping list, an open mind, and a whole bunch of recipes can start you on the journey to Paleolithic successs. Switching over to eating Paleo does not have to be an arduous task. In fact, many of the recipes adored by families the world over can be converted quite simply to Paleo recipes with a few careful choices of ingredients and some fun substitution. Here's an example of a common family favorite—spaghetti and meatballs—that has been converted to Paleo:

Paleo Meatballs and Sauce

These meatballs are so close to the original, you won't know the difference.

INGREDIENTS | **YIELDS 12–14 MEATBALLS**

1 (16-ounce) can diced, no-salt-added tomatoes

1 (4-ounce) can organic, no-salt-added tomato paste

2 pounds grass-fed ground beef

1 cup chopped celery

1 cup chopped onion

1 cup chopped carrots

4 finely chopped garlic cloves

3 eggs

½ cup flaxseed meal

1 tablespoon oregano

1 teaspoon black pepper

¼ teaspoon chili powder

1. Pour canned tomatoes and tomato paste into slow cooker.

2. Place all remaining ingredients in a large bowl and mix well with hands.

3. Roll resulting meat mixture into 2–3 ounce (large, rounded tablespoon) balls and add to slow cooker.

4. Cook on low for 5 hours minimum.

Pasta is a staple in many homes but it is not included in the Paleolithic diet. A fantastic alternative to pasta is spaghetti squash. This amazingly delicious member of the squash family softens when cooked in the oven for less than 45 minutes and with the light touch of a fork, can be pulled to form "strings." Add the Paleo Meatballs and Sauce recipe and you have a perfect, healthy, and 100 percent Paleolithic lifestyle–approved meatball and spaghetti meal.

What Will I Eat?

Back in the Pleistocene Epoch humans ate anything that was in season that they could find or hunt. That included game meat, organ meat, fish, chicken, eggs, fruit, vegetables, root vegetables, nuts, and seeds. There are a huge number of everyday foods that fall within this list. Some of the foods are common: beef, turkey, salmon, swordfish, almonds, avocados, strawberries, apples, spinach, and broccoli. Some of the foods are more obscure: venison, quail, moose, bear, kumquats, ugly fruit, and dandelion leaf. When eating on this plan, it is thought that you do not have to watch exactly what you eat. If you eat various portions of protein, with a vegetable or fruit, and a small amount of fat, you should be satiated and obtain maximum nutritional benefit from your food. This approach does not always work for everyone and will be addressed later in the book.

Although the list of Paleo acceptable foods is long, there are some choices that are more beneficial than others. Foods rich in omega-3 fatty acids promote optimal health and well-being. Some great omega-3 choices include:

PROTEIN SOURCES OF OMEGA-3
- Wild-caught salmon
- Cold water fish such as mackerel, herring, sturgeon
- Free-range poultry
- Grass-fed beef

FAT SOURCES OF OMEGA-3
- Walnuts (particularly black walnuts)
- Brazil nuts
- Flaxseed

CARBOHYDRATE SOURCES OF OMEGA-3
- Broccoli
- Collard greens
- Raspberries
- Strawberries

On the Paleolithic plan, you will want to find fruits and vegetables with lower glycemic levels. These foods will not have a big impact on your blood sugar and insulin levels in your body. By keeping these levels lower and in balance you will promote wellness and reduce any unnecessary inflammation. Foods with lower glycemic levels include:

LOW GLYCEMIC LEVEL FRUITS
- Apple
- Grapefruit
- Kiwi
- Orange
- Pear
- Plum
- Strawberries
- Raspberries

LOW GLYCEMIC LEVEL VEGETABLES
- Asparagus
- Beet greens
- Broccoli
- Cabbage
- Cauliflower
- Celery
- Swiss chard
- Collard greens

For a complete list of acceptable Paleo foods see Appendix A at the end of this book.

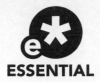

Fiber is defined as the undigestible components of plants. This material helps to maintain good digestion, promotes passage of food through the gastrointestinal tract, and shortens the amount of time food is found in the body. The Paleolithic lifestyle has ample fiber to aid and fix most digestion issues.

Foods to Avoid

Paleolithic hunter-gatherers ate foods that were pre-agricultural. They did not farm the land or herd animals for sustenance. Grains such as wheat, oats, barley, quinoa, and rice were not a part of their diet. Neither were potatoes or legumes of any sort including soybeans and peanuts. When these foods are in their natural, raw state they are toxic for the human body due to the presence of toxins called lectins. Lectins have been linked to many ailments, but predominantly they cause "leaky gut" syndromes in human intestinal tracts.

There are several symptoms of leaky gut syndrome. These symptoms include abdominal discomfort, heartburn, bloating, gluten and food intolerance, muscle cramps, and abdominal pain. In addition to lecithin, diets high in processed foods, low in fiber and nutrients, and with high levels of additives contribute to this disorder. On the Paleolithic diet you would avoid all foods linked to this and many other diseases.

Grains, beans, and potatoes are poor sources of vitamins A, B, folic acid, and C. They have a negative impact on your blood sugar levels causing a spike in insulin released from your pancreas. Additionally, they have low mineral and antioxidant profiles.

Dairy Products

The plight of the dairy industry is alarming. As the farming industry injects livestock with hormones to boost productivity, consumers are slowly but increasingly ingesting it themselves. The pasteurizing and homogenizing practices to sterilize milk are killing proteins in enzymes that are beneficial. Moreover, the claims that the best source of calcium for growing children comes from milk is false. There are many vegetables that are good sources of calcium that can be used in place of milk and milk products.

CALCIUM-RICH FOODS		
Food Source	Serving Size	Calcium (mg)
Broccoli	1 stalk	112
Bok choy	1 cup	158
Dandelion greens	1 cup	147
Collard greens	1 cup	266
Sweet potato	1 cup	89
Kale	1 cup	94
Swiss chard	1 cup	102
Whole milk	1 cup	300

Calcium content data derived from USDA National Nutrient Database for Standard Reference, Release 19

Although it is true that one glass of whole milk has more milligrams of calcium, you can see how it would be easy enough to obtain that same amount from a healthier vegetable source as listed above.

Almost 4 billion people are lactose intolerant due to genetics. Expression of the gene for producing lactase, the enzyme responsible for breaking down milk sugar, declines after age two resulting in the common intestinal ailment.

How to Be Successful on the Paleolithic Diet Plan

As with any lifestyle change, you are sure to be confronted with obstacles along the way. What are you going to eat with your friends? What are you going to cook each day? How are you going to live without soda and popcorn at the movies? This plan is not easy to start, but there are some things that you can implement early on to ease the transition. These few tricks will make this plan seem more manageable, more comfortable, and simply more fun.

Slow Cookers

You can usually find slow cookers where you find most small appliances. These mini ovens are like chefs. They enable you to pack the most flavor into your food and give even the most inexperienced cooks confidence in the kitchen. They are simple to operate and are practically foolproof. And, best of all, you can throw everything in there and leave it for hours at a time. Over the course of several hours your food will absorb the flavorings of spices and vegetables that you didn't know existed. You will feel like a personal chef when you finish a recipe prepared in this magical little invention. Try the following recipe:

Pulled Chicken

This chicken will melt in your mouth after hours in the slow cooker.

INGREDIENTS | SERVES 8

2 pounds barn-roaming chicken breast

1 (16-ounce) can diced tomatoes

1 cup diced sweet onion

4 carrots, cut into large pieces

2 green onions

4 garlic cloves, cut coarsely

1 tablespoon thyme

1 teaspoon chili powder

Combine all ingredients into slow cooker and cook on high for 5 hours. Reduce heat and serve.

The great thing about a slow cooker is you can throw in whatever vegetable or meat that you like. The recipe options are endless. They are great for desserts as well. For more great slow cooker recipes, see the recipe chapters in the book.

Storage and Cooking in Bulk

An important component of being successful is in the planning. It is critical that you shop and cook in large amounts and store meals in containers for the future. Otherwise, you will be cooking around the clock and feel overwhelmed. The best idea would be to develop a routine where you cook three or four meals together and store in the refrigerator or freezer.

ALERT

Bisphenol A, otherwise known as BPA, is an organic compound used in some plastic products. This chemical may be linked to neurological and brain development issues in fetuses and infants. Be sure to find plastic storage products that are marked BPA-free or use glass storage containers for bulk food items.

Track Your Success

The Paleolithic lifestyle is sure to bring about drastic changes in your body and health. All of your successes should be recorded. A daily log book where you can record your progress and changes will serve as the most motivation you will ever need. Use a book to record:

- ❏ Daily meals
- ❏ How you are feeling (hungry, satiated, and so on)
- ❏ Exercise and performance
- ❏ Recipes found
- ❏ Recipes used
- ❏ Current weight
- ❏ Body fat changes
- ❏ Performance goals
- ❏ Body change goals

Not only will this book serve as a motivator, but it will track the changes you have made along the journey. It's hard to remember where you have come from and this will serve as a reminder of the old, unhealthy you. Remember, no journey worth traveling is easy and converting over to the Paleolithic lifestyle is no exception. Rest assured, it will be worth it.

CHAPTER 2

Wellness and
the Paleolithic Diet

The positive health benefits of eating as your Paleolithic ancestors ate are plentiful. Body fat will be reduced, overall weight will normalize, you will feel better than you have in years, and your body will be internally healthy. Often times, sickness in the body goes unnoticed. Your body has a way of masking pain with natural pain relievers. Living as your Paleolithic ancestors did will help to fight off the smaller, unnoticeable issues that you have learned to ignore. You will look good and feel good as a result. You will need less over-the-counter and prescription medication. You will spring out of bed in the morning with your eyes wide open instead of needing a jolt of caffeine before you can converse with someone. These are only a few of the wellness benefits the Paleolithic lifestyle will provide.

Health Benefits of the Paleolithic Lifestyle

If you take a look at the last remaining hunter-gatherer tribes on this earth, you will find no heart disease, high cholesterol, obesity, or diabetes. What you will find are a conditioned, muscular, aerobically active group of people that are light years more healthy and fit overall. What do they have or know that you do not? According to Loren Cordain, author of *The Paleo Diet*, more than 50 percent of adult Americans over the age of twenty-five are obese. Additionally, childhood obesity rates have risen to epidemic proportions. The obesity rate in children aged six to eleven has gone from 6.5 percent to 19.6 percent over twenty years and teenage obesity rates have more than tripled from 5 percent in 1980 to 18.1 percent in 2008.

The current situation is alarming and steps to remedy these issues must start with the diet. The Paleolithic lifestyle will naturally bring your body into balance and obesity issues will not be a problem. It will lower your cholesterol levels, blood glucose levels, and solve hypertension issues without medication. If you eat what your genetics dictate, you will find the maximum health that you long for.

Silent Inflammation

Inflammation to the level that one feels pain is common. Silent inflammation is unnoticed inflammation and is more detrimental because it goes undetected, often for long periods of time. Three hormones—cortisol, insulin, and eicosanoids—contribute to silent inflammation in your body, but with some simple Paleolithic diet techniques, your levels can be stabilized to reduce the inflammatory response.

Eicosanoids

This hormone is produced in every cell in your body and its main function is to work with your immune system to help you fight invaders. There are two types in your body. One helps as an anti-inflammatory to reduce inflammation in your body. The other works to help destroy tissue and acts as a pro-inflammatory. Your body needs both to function normally, but they need to be in balance; not too much of one over the other.

There is a direct link between eicosanoid hormone production and fatty acid consumption. Pro-inflammatory eicosanoids are made with the help of omega-6 fatty acids. In cases where a person eats more omega-6 over the anti-inflammatory omega-3 fatty acids, their inflammatory eicosanoids will be higher, thus contributing to silent inflammation. To increase the amount of the better hormone, a diet rich in omega-3 fatty acids over a diet richer in omega-6 fatty acids is best. The Paleolithic diet naturally encourages a diet higher in omega-3.

Insulin

Insulin is the hormone that your body sends out when carbohydrates or sugar enters the bloodstream. Its function is to allow glucose to be taken up by cells in the liver and muscles. If that energy is not used right away it will be stored as glycogen, a complex carbohydrate molecule, in those cells. The more sugar that someone eats, the more insulin will be released to deal with it. Greater insulin increases the production of a substance found to be directly related to pro-inflammatory eicosanoid formation. As stated previously, this contributes significantly to silent inflammation.

Data from the 2007 National Diabetes Fact Sheet states that 23.6 million children and adults in the United States have diabetes. That is 7.8 percent of the entire U.S. population. It is listed as the seventh leading cause of death in the United States.

Cortisol

Cortisol, sometimes referred to as your flight or fight hormone, is produced by the adrenal glands. When your body is in a stressed condition this hormone is released to deal with the stress. It does that by trying to diminish the eicosanoid hormones. According to Dr. Barry Sears, author of *The Zone*, this causes insulin resistance. Insulin resistance tapers back your immune response and, in turn, can make you sicker.

Insulin Resistance

When a large surge of carbohydrate is ingested, the body produces a large amount of insulin to prevent the excess blood sugar. This actually can produce a dip in blood sugar level that is below average. In response to that dip, you release cortisol and adrenaline (another powerful hormone in your body). After each episode of eating large carbohydrates, this same procedure happens: big release of insulin, big dip below average of blood sugar levels in response to the insulin, then release of cortisol and adrenaline. This up-and-down pattern can lead to a condition known as insulin resistance. Insulin resistance often leads to type-2 diabetes, a disease where the body ignores the insulin that is released, thus sugar is not taken up by the cells for energy use.

All Fats Are Not Created Equal

Fats have gotten a bad rap in diets today. Most people trying to lose weight would say to avoid them at all cost. Fats, however, are incredibly beneficial and important in your diet. According to a recent study published in the *American Journal of Clinical Nutrition*, fats are not only good to have, but are necessary for vitamin and nutrient absorption. The important differentiation is in the type of fat you consume. Saturated fats, those that are solid at room temperatures, are the type that clog arteries and promote heart disease. Unsaturated fats, those that are liquid at room temperature, are completely different in their structure and impact on the human body. These types of fats protect you from illness and disease.

QUESTION

What is the fatty acid ratio of commercially grain-fed beef to grass-fed beef?
Grass-fed beef has a ratio of omega-6 to omega-3 of 1.65 versus 4.84 for grain-fed beef. In addition, it is higher in vitamin E, thiamin, riboflavin, calcium, potassium, and magnesium, and is lower in saturated fat and overall fat content.

Essential Fatty Acids

There are two essential fatty acids that must be attained in the diet: alpha linoleic acid, an omega-3 fatty acid, and linoleic acid, an omega-6 fatty acid. The way in which these two fatty acids interact with each other is very important. One, omega-3 fatty acid, has an anti-inflammatory response. The other, omega-6, has a pro-inflammatory response. Both of these responses are needed in the body, but the careful balance of them is critical in a well-functioning body. If the ratio of omega-6 to omega-3 is not low—low being around 2 or 3 to 1—you promote inflammation, heart disease, autoimmune diseases. The diets of today promote an unfavorably high omega-6 to omega-3 ratio. Our ancestors from the Paleolithic time period had ratios of omega-6 to omega-3 of about 3 to 1, while today's average ratios are 10 to 1 or higher.

ALERT

It is critically important that babies get enough omega-3 fatty acids from their mothers during pregnancy or run the risk of developing vision and nerve problems.

Benefits of Omega-3 Fatty Acids

The incredible list of health benefits of omega-3 fatty acids is ever increasing. Currently, this essential fatty acid is found to be beneficial at fighting the following diseases:

- Heart disease
- Inflammation
- Irritable bowel syndrome
- High cholesterol
- High blood pressure
- Diabetes
- Rheumatoid arthritis
- Lupus
- Osteoporosis
- Depression

- Bipolar disorder
- Attention deficit hyperactivity disorder
- Asthma
- Cancer

ALERT

One of the benefits of omega-3 is the ability to thin the blood and counteract blood clotting. It should be taken with caution when used in conjunction with blood-thinning medication.

Foods Rich in Omega-3

There are three types of omega-3 fatty acids that can be found in foods: EPA, DHA, and ALA. EPA, or eicosapentaenoic acid, and DHA, docosahexaenoic acid, are found in cold-water fish such as:

- Wild-caught salmon
- Mackerel
- Halibut
- Sardines
- Tuna
- Herring

Good sources of ALA, or alpha-linoleic acid, are:

- Flaxseed
- Flaxseed oil
- Canola (rapeseed) oil
- Pumpkin seeds
- Walnuts
- Walnut oil

If eating foods with ample omega-3 content is difficult, there are several fish oil supplements on the market. They can be found in liquid or capsule form. The liquid form is best for maximum absorption, but the capsules will provide adequate EFAs. When shopping for a capsule supplement, look for the highest amount of EPA and DHA available per capsule to ensure you are getting the same benefits as consuming the essential fatty acids in food.

Other Beneficial Fatty Acids

Omega-3 is not the only fatty acid needed by the body. Omega-6 fatty acid can be found in many plant-based oils such as evening primrose oil, borage oil, and black currant seed oil. These oils can help to reduce inflammation and are important for the body. Remember, the most important thing to consider is the ratio of omega-6 to omega-3. It is ideal to keep the ratios of these two fatty acids around three or four to one. Omega-9 is not an essential fatty acid as it is produced in the body. If there is a shortage of omega-3 or omega-6, your body will try to convert omega-9 to the other fatty acids. This is not an effective way to obtain these essential fatty acids and it will be detrimental to your health in the long term.

Superfoods

If someone told you that there are foods that have undeniable health benefits, ward off illness, and put you in a better mood, would you eat them? Superfoods do exist and they are easily accessible and encouraged on the Paleolithic lifestyle plan. These foods will boost your immune system and provide you more nutrient-packed power than normal food items.

Spirulina

Spirulina is a tiny blue-green alga that lives in warm, alkaline fresh waters. The nutritional profile of this little organism surpasses red meat. It is made up of 60 to 70 percent complete protein. This means that spirulina contains every amino acid your body needs to build muscle and produce proteins. Additionally, spirulina contains more vitamins and minerals than most land plants. This superfood may be taken as a supplement, but also can be used in cooking. Following is a great spirulina recipe:

Vegan Spirulina Pesto

This quick and easy spirulina recipe can be eaten immediately. Just blend up and enjoy.

INGREDIENTS | **SERVES 2**

2 cups organic basil
1 cup ground/powdered white sesame seeds
½ cup no-salt beef broth
1 teaspoon almond butter
1 clove garlic
1–1½ cups water
¼ teaspoon spirulina

1. Cut off stems and wash basil.

2. Grind sesame seeds in coffee grinder into a powder.

3. Add all dry ingredients to blender. Blend, adding water gradually to desired consistency.

4. Turn off blender then add spirulina powder to desired color.

Goji

The goji berry, otherwise known as the wolfberry, has been used for its medicinal properties as well as food for many years, although it has recently gained popularity as its superfood qualities are discovered. It is native to southeastern Europe and Asia and is primarily imported from China. This fruit contains eleven essential minerals, six essential vitamins, eighteen amino acids, and five fatty acids, including linoleic and alpha-linoleic acid. It is usually sold in its dried form, but does not contain the high glycemic levels that other dried fruits such as raisins or dates have. It has a sweet taste, is especially great for snacking, and is a perfect food for adding to trail mix.

Cacao

Cacao comes from a dried and fermented fatty seed of Theobroma (which means food of the gods) cacao bean. Cacao is a rich source of flavonoids and contains more antioxidant properties than blueberries, goji berries, and green tea. Prolonged use of raw cacao and its high flavonoid antioxidants has been linked to cardiovascular health benefits. Cacao can be used in cooking and eaten whole in the raw. Many Paleo enthusiasts use cacao to make sweet baked goods such as the recipe listed here:

Paleo Cacao Nib Cookies

If you are looking for a sweet treat try these Paleo cookies. These can be taken anywhere on the go and will give you satisfaction for your sweet tooth cravings.

INGREDIENTS | YIELDS 24 COOKIES

1 cup almond butter
⅔ cup shredded coconut
1½ tablespoons coconut oil
½ cup almond butter
1 cup cacao nibs
⅓ cup coconut flour
½ teaspoon cinnamon
1 egg
2 tablespoons cacao powder
½ cup raw honey

1. Combine all ingredients into a large mixing bowl.

2. Spoon rounded teaspoon-sized balls onto a cookie sheet sprayed with nonstick cooking spray.

3. Cook for 9 minutes at 350°F.

Walnuts

Walnuts are an exemplary superfood because they were the first recognized superfood by the U.S. Food and Drug Administration. These nuts are a superior source of alpha-linoleic acid, an essential omega-3 fatty acid, which has been shown to aid in all types of heart disease and other illnesses. Walnuts can be purchased whole or as an oil and are a great addition to baked goods, salads, and side dish recipes.

FACT

All nuts are not created equal. Most commercially sold nuts have a very high omega-6 to omega-3 fatty acid ratio. Almonds, in particular, are quite high. Walnuts provide the best ratio around 4:1.

Berries

It has been known for a while that berries have high antioxidant properties. The more antioxidants you eat, the better chance you have to fight heart disease and free radicals in your body. In a study published in the *Journal of Agricultural and Food Chemistry* it was shown that berries, namely cranberries, blueberries, and blackberries, ranked among the highest of the fruits studied. As a general rule, the more colorful the fruit or vegetable, the better the antioxidant capabilities. It is always best to eat a variety of foods with a plethora of colors to promote the best fight against free radical oxidation in your body.

FACT

Although the debate is still out as to wheat grass as a superfood, it has been shown that a diet high in chlorophyll level, those items that are dark green in color, can lead to lower rates of colon cancer.

Benefits of Coconut Products

The real benefits of coconut are just being made more public. For a long time, coconut got a bad reputation due to its high saturated fat content. More recently, however, it has come to the forefront that coconut has many beneficial properties that are not only good nutritionally, but medicinally as well. Coconut is made up of a unique type of fatty acid characterized as a medium chain triglyceride. Medium chain triglycerides do not raise blood cholesterol levels and do not contribute to heart disease.

FACT

Coconut oil is an effective anti-viral, antibacterial, and anti-fungal. It has been used to help people suffering from thyroid and metabolism issues and to lose weight. Additionally, it has been shown to help fight cancer.

Various Coconut Products

There are several parts of the coconut that can be eaten. The inside of the coconut is filled with sterile coconut water that is high in fiber, vitamins, minerals, antioxidants, protein, and sugar. This water is a great source of electrolytes and is the perfect post-workout drink when mixed with a protein source. Coconut meat comes from the fleshy part of the nut and can be eaten dried or fresh. Coconut milk is a liquid that can be squeezed from coconut meat. The oil can be extracted from the nut and used in cooking and baking. Due to its recent popularity, coconut oil can be found at your local produce or vitamin supplement store. Below is a great coconut recipe that is perfect for post workout:

Power Packed Protein Shake

This shake will restore glycogen storage and provide your body with amino acids to rebuild torn tissue.

INGREDIENTS | **SERVES 1**

1 tablespoon coconut oil

8 ounces coconut water

1 scoop protein powder of choice

Add all ingredients to a blender and blend until combined completely.

Coconut is a favorite when baking Paleolithic treats. Its consistency provides a good base flour for any cookie or cake-like recipe. Try the following coconut recipe when you are craving something sweet:

Coconut Cacao Cookies

When you're craving a sweet chocolate treat, try these coconut cacao cookies. They are quick and satisfying.

INGREDIENTS | **YIELDS 12–14 COOKIES**

7 pitted dates
¾ cup almond flour
¼ cup coconut flour
½ cup shredded, unsweetened coconut
1 teaspoon coconut oil
2 tablespoons coconut milk
1 egg
1 cup cacao nibs

1. Combine dates and unsweetened coconut into food processor and pulse until crumb-like consistency.

2. Pour mixture into a large mixing bowl and add remaining ingredients. Mix well with hands.

3. Form into patties and place on baking sheet sprayed with nonstick cooking spray.

4. Bake at 350°F for 22 minutes.

Coconut oil is particularly good for sautéing food as it has a very high melting temperature. A nice way to cook vegetables with coconut oil is to steam them first in water just shy of becoming soft, then transfer over to the sauté pan and cook in oil. It will reduce your time for cooking and will not sauté all the nutrients out of the vegetables. Coconut oil is particularly nice for quick searing and stir-frying.

CHAPTER 3

Paleolithic Lifestyle and Performance

Everyone wants to be faster, stronger, and more athletic. The Paleolithic diet can truly increase athletic performance and unleash gains in human potential not seen previously with other diets. The Paleo lifestyle gives the body the fuel it needs to increase health and decrease recovery time. Those two aspects alone make a transition over to this lifestyle more than worthwhile.

Increased Athletic Performance

There are those who believe that an athlete's potential is in their genetics. That is true to some extent. Genetic predisposition for certain sports cannot be denied. For example, height contributing to a basketball player's success or a sprinter's percentage of fast twitch versus slow twitch muscle fibers. A taller athlete may have an easier time getting the ball in the basket and an athlete with more fast twitch muscle fibers will most likely be able to run faster for a short burst than a person with a greater number of slow twitch muscle fibers. Although these genetic advantages must be acknowledged, there is a great deal of benefit that your diet can play in your athletic performance. For years the traditional pasta "loading" meal the night before the event has been served. And, in concept, it is not completely inaccurate. However, pasta as a source of energy for athletes is not the best choice. Some better Paleo friendly alternatives could come from vegetables, fruit, squashes, and sweet potatoes. These choices will provide better results than those heavy pasta meals. The traditional type of loading options will wreak havoc on your hormones and cause a great deal of silent inflammation in your body. On race day, you do not need anything further to deal with than the exertion your body will undergo from the race.

ALERT

Sweet potatoes are often considered to be a no-no by many Paleolithic enthusiasts. These starchy potatoes are packed with great vitamins and minerals and are a very good choice for pre- and post-workout fuel due to their lower glycemic carbohydrate load. They are packed with vitamins A, C, and B_6 and have more potassium than a banana, a common choice for athletes. Additionally, sweet potatoes are highly anti-inflammatory, a topic of great importance when discussing overall well-being.

Blood Sugar Level Balance

For an athlete, blood sugar level balance is a major concern. In fact, it should be a major concern for everyone, whether an athlete or not. In order for your body to fuel and power itself, it must have access to an energy source. The most efficient source for your body to metabolize is from carbohydrates and they are stored primarily in your muscles and liver in the form of a molecule called glycogen. Understanding the way glycogen is made and used in the body will give you a better idea as to how important it is to regulate its balance.

Insulin and Glucagon

As a meal containing carbohydrates is eaten it is absorbed through the walls of the small intestine where it enters the bloodstream. When the levels of carbohydrates (sugar) increase in the blood it triggers the release of insulin from the pancreas into the bloodstream, as well. Insulin is the hormone that deals with the synthesis of glycogen in the liver. As insulin reaches the liver and detects the presence of the sugar, it initiates sugar molecules to stick together like Legos. This Lego-type structure is the glycogen. It is being made for later use by the body. Once the sugar levels in the blood decrease, the production of insulin in the pancreas also decreases, which, in turn, stops the synthesizing of the glycogen chains. Alternatively, when glycogen is needed by the body to do work, another hormone, glucagon, is secreted by the pancreas. This hormone initiates the breaking down of glycogen into sugar molecules again for the body to use to power itself. Together these two hormones, insulin and glucagon, control the storage and release of carbohydrates in the body. They are extremely necessary and powerful chemicals that every human body depends on. Without them you would not have the ability to store energy or release it when needed for activity.

FACT

Insulin has many functions that are helpful to an athlete. It inhibits the breakdown of stored fats so that you use carbohydrates, the more efficient energy source. Insulin also inhibits protein breakdown and stimulates protein synthesis, so muscle fibers that are used can be rebuilt.

Balancing Act

When your body needs energy, insulin and glucagon are responsible for controlling what source gets used. The key for any athlete is to know how much to fuel themselves so that they have the right amount needed to perform the task at hand, without excess. Your body will use only what it needs and will store the rest for that "rainy day" or starvation period. That is when weight gain appears. The trick to controlling weight gain and body-fat increases is to find out what level of energy your body needs to sustain itself. The more exercise you exert, the more energy that is needed. The more energy that is needed, the more important it is for you to control your hormones. Excess hormones in response to excess energy needs are what cause imbalances in hormone levels. That, in turn, will lead to mood swings, "sugar highs" and eventual crashes, energy disruptions during exercise, and feelings of light-headedness.

Paleolithic Lifestyle and Athletes

Just as your Paleolithic ancestors were exercising to find their next meal, the Paleo lifestyle is particularly good for athletes. This plan promotes a balance in hormone levels by eating foods relatively low in glycemic value. Fresh fruits and vegetables provide you with an adequate amount of carbohydrates while not overloading the body with unnecessary sugars from high–glycemic load choices such as starches, grains, and beans.

Exceptions to the Rule

Of course, not all plans are 100 percent foolproof and the Paleolithic lifestyle is no exception. There may be times when it is beneficial for you to use higher–glycemic index carbohydrate items for fuel. Since it is optimal for an athlete to use glycogen to power exercise, if the exercise you are performing is particularly strenuous and depletes all storage or there is not enough storage to begin with, you must fuel or refuel your body accordingly.

QUESTION

Can I use natural forms of sugar before or after a workout?
In the strict Paleo lifestyle, the only form of sugar that is acceptable is natural honey. This may be used as a form of energy before, after, or during an event if needed. Additionally, as an exception to strict Paleo, sport gels have been used quite effectively among endurance athletes.

Pre- and Post-Event or Workout Nutrition

Before and after a race or workout it is of critical importance to give your body what it will need to function to its potential while exerting itself. That is where careful pre- and post-workout nutrition comes into play. If you do not adhere to fueling your body, it will fail or break down when you do not want it to. An occasional bad fueling will not be harmful, but the repetitive decision to not give your body what it needs will cause injuries and illness to prevail.

Pre-Workout Nutrition

The food that you eat before a workout is to fuel your body for the event it's about to do. This type of fuel needs to be light, relatively quick assimilating, and produce a lower insulin response to avoid a spike in hormones and thus a crash during your workout. A meal that contains some good fat, lean protein, and low glycemic carbohydrates is best.

GOOD PRE-WORKOUT FUEL SOURCES		
Protein	**Fat**	**Carbohydrate**
Tuna	Avocado	Strawberries
White meat chicken	Flax oil	Blueberries
White meat turkey	Uddo's oil	Apple
Tilapia	Seeds	Grapefruit
Cod	Nuts	Raspberries

Once you have completed an athletic event, it is extremely important to refuel your body and provide it with the necessary ingredients to recover. During a race or long workout your body uses its glycogen storage and breaks down muscle fibers. Your job postworkout is to supply your body with the necessary building blocks to reconstruct muscle and store glycogen once again. The two food groups that are most useful at this time are protein and carbohydrate. Additionally, it might be necessary to rehydrate and replace lost electrolytes. A meal containing a lean protein source and a higher-glycemic carbohydrate is a perfect recovery meal. Fat, post workout, is not necessary and is best left for a meal two or more hours after the post-workout meal.

GOOD POST-WORKOUT FUEL SOURCES	
Protein	**Carbohydrate**
Whey protein	Sweet potato
White meat chicken	No-sugar-added applesauce
Tilapia	Mango
Shrimp	Melon
White meat turkey	Grapes

Fueling Your Body During an Event or Race

According to the website *www.exrx.net*, the average person stores enough glycogen to last them twelve to fourteen hours or more than two hours with sustained moderate intensity. That being said, there will be times on longer-endurance workouts or events that you will need to refuel your body. As a general rule, any workout longer than ninety minutes will require a small protein, carbohydrate, and fat combination snack. This should be easily transportable and small enough to fit on you while working out. The following recipe is a nice option:

Quick and Easy Protein Power Balls

This recipe is a perfect food for during an event. It is small, easily transported, and tastes great.

INGREDIENTS | **YIELDS 8–10 BALLS (35 CALORIES EACH)**

1 banana
2 tablespoons almond butter
1 scoop chocolate whey protein powder

1. Mash banana and combine with almond butter and whey protein. If consistency is not thick, add more whey protein powder.

2. Using a tablespoon, scoop batter into palm and round into balls.

3. Store in refrigerator or freezer for later use.

The mainstream guideline for fueling during endurance workouts is roughly 300 calories per hour. Each power ball contains approximately thirty-five calories, thus eight to nine balls would be sufficient energy per hour.

ESSENTIAL

During an athletic event you lose electrolytes in your sweat. One important electrolyte, sodium, is needed for proper functioning of muscle contraction and nervous system control. A quick and easy way to increase sodium before a race is to eat a pickle. The amount of salt in the pickle will give you just the right amount of sodium you will need to maintain good muscular movement and quick reaction timing.

Recovery from Athletic Events

When thinking about recovery from an athletic event you should be considering the time period an hour or two after the event is over. During this time it is beneficial to have foods rich in omega-3 fatty acids to decrease inflammation and aid in recovery of tissue. Foods high in omega-3 include:

- Wild-caught salmon
- Grass-fed beef
- Walnuts
- Flaxseed
- Sardines
- Flax oil

Vitamins and minerals in fruits and vegetables are particularly important now to aid in repair. Vitamin C is a very powerful antioxidant and helps to repair damaged tissue in the body. Good sources of vitamin C include:

- Red pepper
- Kale
- Broccoli

- Kiwi
- Green pepper
- Cantaloupe

FACT

Vitamin C helps to fight cancer, regenerate vitamin E sources, and protect from free-radical oxidation in your body. Contrary to popular belief, citrus fruits are not the best sources of vitamin C. There is more vitamin C in a papaya or red pepper than an orange or grapefruit.

When you exercise you increase the formation of free radicals in your body. Antioxidants such as vitamin C and E are known to fight against free radicals that are released from damaged tissues during exercise. Some sources of vitamin E can be found in:

- Pine nuts
- Sunflower seeds
- Vegetable and fish oils
- Avocado
- Apricots

Minerals are important in your body in many capacities. Magnesium, for example, is imperative in muscle and nervous tissue function. This mineral can be found in green vegetables such as spinach, kale, and mustard greens. Zinc is a mineral that is good for protein synthesis. It can be found in beef, liver, sesame, pumpkin, and sunflower seeds, alfalfa, celery, and almonds.

Eat Like an Olympic Athlete

Eating to better your performance is one thing. Eating like an Olympian is a whole different category. This level of athleticism requires discipline that most of the average world does not comprehend. Nutrition, rest, and recovery must be 100 percent on point. If you want to see incredible gains in your athletic ability, you must plan all your meals and weigh and measure every morsel to ensure the correct amount of macronutrients. Your body will need fuel, stored energy, and building blocks to recover adequately and prepare itself for the next athletic event.

Sample Athlete Macronutrient Values

The standard on protein consumption, according to athletic coach and nutritionist Jodi Jones of Modelper4mance.com, is 1.25 to 2.0 grams of protein per pound of lean body mass (lean body mass being the key terms here). It is inefficient to feed parts of your body that cannot process the protein, so you are only interested in fueling and sparing the lean muscle that you have. As a general rule on fat consumption, most men need about fifty grams of good fat per day while women need about forty grams. To determine the rest of the macronutrients, you must look at the activity level of the athlete and their total caloric consumption needs. There are two formulas that can be used to determine daily total caloric intake. One is called the Harris Benedict Equation and the other is the Katch McArdle. Both of these equations use an athlete's basal metabolic rate, but the Katch McArdle takes into account an athlete's lean muscle mass, which is the part of the body you want to fuel. For that reason, this calculator is more accurate and better when referencing athlete's nutrition.

KATCH MCARDLE EQUATION
Basal Metabolic Rate = 370 + (21.6 × lean mass in Kg)
Conversion from pounds to Kg = pounds ÷ 2.2

Katch, Frank, Katch, Victor, McArdle, William. *Exercise Physiology: Energy, Nutrition, and Human Performance, 4th edition*. Williams & Wilkins, 1996.

ACTIVITY FACTOR	
Level of Exertion	**Activity Factor**
Sedentary/little or no exercise	1.2
Lightly active/exercise 1–3 days/week	1.375
Moderately active/exercise 3–5 days/week	1.55
Very active/hard exercise 6–7 days/week	1.725
Extra active/very hard daily exercise	1.9

Katch, Frank, Katch, Victor, McArdle, William. *Exercise Physiology: Energy, Nutrition, and Human Performance, 4th edition*. Williams & Wilkins, 1996.

Putting It All Together

Once you have determined your lean body mass you can put it all together and determine your ideal daily macronutrient values. This is the first step in really organizing your diet to fueling your body. Once you determine these values, you can start to have fun with menu planning. Partitioning daily values throughout your day is an intelligent and precise way to fuel your body and obtain peak performance. Food is not just to make you happy anymore. It is to power a streamlined and efficient machine—YOU! Below are sample macronutrient values for a typical man and woman.

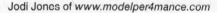

SAMPLE MACRONUTRIENT TABLE FOR "LIGHTLY ACTIVE" INDIVIDUALS					
200-pound Male 15% Bodyfat			**140-pound Female 20% Bodyfat**		
Calculated BMR = 2,040 calories			Calculated BMR = 1,470 calories		
Activity factor = 1.375			Activity factor = 1.375		
Protein	**Fat**	**Carb**	**Protein**	**Fat**	**Carb**
213g	50g	242g	140g	40g	178g
935cal	450cal	1065cal	616cal	360cal	784cal
38%	18%	44%	35%	20%	45%

Jodi Jones of *www.modelper4mance.com*

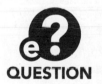

QUESTION

What type of protein is best?
When choosing protein options it is best to stay on the leaner side. Examples of lean proteins are white meat chicken, white meat turkey, extra lean (99 percent fat free) ground meats, egg whites, and white fishes. That does not mean that you must eat lean choices all the time, but aim for 80 percent adherence if your goal is to increase lean body mass and lose body fat.

Snacks "On the Go"

It's important to remember that eating every few hours keeps your metabolism roaring. As an athlete, the demands on your body will be larger than the average person. Luckily, this comes with the added benefit of being able to eat more. The downside is that you must fuel your body more often. For some, this will be a tough transition. However, this does not have to be an arduous task. The trick is to keep quick and easy snacks with you at all times.

QUESTION

What is a good, quick, on-the-go snack that I can have during the day?
It's more important that you know to constantly fuel your body. But, if you look at those athletes who do fuel often, you will see a strong and healthy competitor. A quick meal of organic, no-salt-added turkey jerky, walnuts, cacao nibs, and mulberries can be thrown in a plastic baggie and eaten anywhere at anytime.

Supplementation

Strict Paleo eaters do not use any supplements of any kind. As an athlete, however, it is acceptable and often necessary to incorporate a few good choices. One such example is the addition of a good protein shake into your diet. A 100 percent whey protein supplement drink without any additives is a great choice. Another would be an egg white protein mix, which is considered Paleo approved. There are several powdered varieties on the market in an array of flavors. They are easily transported and quickly mixed with water or coconut water. The most important factor to consider when choosing a protein powder is to get one that has a relatively low carbohydrate value (three grams or fewer) and low-fat value (two grams or fewer) per serving. A full serving of protein would be twenty to twenty-four grams per serving.

CHAPTER 4

A Family Affair

Deciding to switch over your lifestyle to eat as your ancestors is not an easy task if you have a family. The Paleolithic lifestyle does not have to be done in seclusion while everyone else in the family is eating high glycemic–loading carbohydrates such as pizza and spaghetti. In fact, that is not recommended. The way to be most successful is enrolling the entire family into the plan. The Paleolithic lifestyle will work for your family with a little planning. When children open the refrigerator and see the plethora of color and variety they will get excited for the flavors they will taste. When the heavenly aroma of fresh herbs and spices fill the house, your loved ones will wonder what new recipe you have concocted for suppertime. Eating Paleo is best implemented when it involves everyone.

Benefits of Paleolithic Lifestyle in Children

Of course any good parent would be concerned about putting their children on a "diet." The Paleolithic lifestyle is not a diet. It is not calorically limiting. It does not leave people feeling hungry and deprived. A true Paleolithic follower eats bountiful macronutrients in the form of protein, carbohydrates, and fat. Post-agricultural dieters also eat all three macronutrients, but the percentages favor refined sugar and high glycemic load carbohydrates that cause massive fluctuation in insulin levels and are poor contributors to healthy macronutrients. The secret to good nutrition for your family is not from grains, dairy, and legumes. It is in the vast array of Paleolithic choices chockfull of vitamins and minerals that your children and family need.

Increase in Refined Sugars

In the past forty years, the amount of refined sugar in the Westernized diet has increased astronomically. Is it a coincidence that the rate of illness has increased as well? The following table shows a trend in sugar consumption that is alarming.

REFINED SUGAR CONSUMPTION IN KG			
Year	Sucrose	High-Fructose Corn Syrup	Glucose
1970	48.2	.2	8.6
1980	37.9	8.8	8.9
1990	29.2	22.5	9.9
2000	29.8	28.9	9.9

American Journal of Clinical Nutrition, Vol. 81, No. 2, 341–354, February 2005, *Origins and Evolution of the Western Diet: Health Implications for the Twenty-First Century,* Loren Cordain, S. Boyd Eaton, Anthony Sebastian, Neil Mann, Staffan Lindeberg, Bruce A. Watkins, James H. O'Keefe, and Janette Brand-Miller.

It is clearly shown in the preceding table that refined sugar consumption has increased overall from 57 Kg in 1970 to more than 68.6 Kg in 2000. More interestingly, the amount of high-fructose corn syrup consumption has tripled. High-fructose corn syrup, often referred to as maize syrup, is derived from corn. It was first developed in 1957 for three main reasons:

- It is about as sweet as table sugar.
- It is cheaper in the United States as a result of corn subsidies by the government and sugar tariffs placed on sucrose.
- Because it is liquid at room temperature, it is easy to blend and transport.

According to the Environmental Working Group and the *New York Times,* the United States government spent $41.9 billion on corn subsidies from 1995 to 2004. This could be a major contributing factor as to how high-fructose corn syrup took over the sugar market in the United States.

High-fructose corn syrup can be found in many items around the super-market. It is added to soft drinks, fruit juice, condiments, processed snacks, bars, ice cream, frozen yogurt, cereal, canned fruit, bread and bread products, and canned soup. It sneaks into places you would not expect like mustard, salad dressing, peanut butter, frozen meals, and deli meats. If you look at the typical child's diet, high-fructose corn syrup is rampant. This sugar is not the kind of carbohydrate your child needs to fuel them. This type of sugar will spike their blood sugar and then immediately cause a crash as insulin tirelessly works to get the blood sugar levels normalized. This will lead to mood swings, hunger pangs, and attention issues as they fight to stay awake.

Mood Swings and Blood Sugar Levels

If you have a young child at home you know about mood swings. Children of all ages have varying moods that can, at times, be challenging to the adults around them. Mood swings have been directly linked to insulin and blood sugar levels. If your child's blood sugar is going up and down, so will their mood. Diabetes, the most common blood sugar imbalance disease in the world today, lists mood swings as a frequent symptom of the disorder. This, too, is because of their increase and decrease of blood sugar levels.

What are good snack choices for my kids that will not spike their insulin?
An easy way to successfully maintain good insulin and blood sugar levels throughout the day for children is to choose a snack that contains all three macronutrients: protein, fat, and carbohydrate. An apple with almond butter or organic, no-salt-added turkey jerky trail mix with added nuts and goji berries are both great balanced choices.

Foods the Entire Family Will Love

You are ready to try the Paleolithic lifestyle, but you are unsure what to serve your family. The first step is to shop. If shopping with the family is an option, it will help to identify the foods your family will enjoy. Bringing the family to the local organic produce store is a great place to start. These stores are full of colorful and unusual fruits and vegetables and fragrant herbs and spices. You will usually find a grass-fed or organic meat department with nice, lower-fat meat selections. Additionally, you will have the advantage of having a bulk section that will likely contain a vast array of nuts, oils, and superfoods such as spirulina, wheat grass, goji berries, mulberries, and cacao. The best part of a mostly organic store is you can rest assured that you can find no-salt-added variety items, and high-fructose corn syrup items are excluded. If it is your first time, bring a shopping list. This will curtail the anxiety of not knowing what to purchase. Some great food items for those with young children include:

- Apples
- Oranges
- Strawberries
- Raspberries
- Grapes
- Bananas
- Broccoli

- Asparagus
- Tomatoes
- Romaine lettuce
- Cucumber
- Carrots
- Red peppers
- Lemons
- Sweet potatoes
- Spaghetti squash
- Free-range chicken
- Grass-fed ground beef
- Cage-free eggs
- Salmon
- Olive oil
- Flax oil
- Nut butter of choice
- Avocado
- Walnuts
- Cacao nibs
- Goji berries
- Organic, no-sugar-added applesauce
- Cans of no-salt-added diced tomatoes or tomato paste
- Dried spices, such as thyme, black pepper, chili powder, oregano, basil
- Fresh spices, such as dill, rosemary, cilantro, parsley, basil

The list above hits all the basics: fruits, vegetables, lean proteins, and good fats but also adds in the items you need to keep it fresh and exciting. Dried spices and fresh herbs will add flavor to the proteins and sauces. Lemon can be used to spice up any dish. Rotating fruits and vegetables around from day to day will help reduce boredom and is best for getting the full benefit of vitamin and mineral profiles. Sweet potato and squashes will help to satiate children who are used to eating high carbohydrate choices. By no means is this list complete and it will not satisfy the tastes of every family. It is merely a starting point.

Paleolithic Lifestyle Beyond the Home

When considering a lifestyle change it is difficult to imagine all the ways in which it will affect you. You do not live in a bubble. You interact with people outside of your home, at school, and at your workplace. It is important to find a way to make the Paleolithic lifestyle work in all those situations or you will feel unsuccessful once you leave your home. Planning and preparation are crucial. Making and preparing foods in advance and transporting them to your work or school will become commonplace. Invest in a good set of plastic containers with lids and lunchboxes for yourself and your children. As long as you are prepared in advance with food and the ability to transport it, you will be successful outside of your home.

Family Gatherings

Family gatherings with non-Paleo eaters do not need to be stressful or difficult. Paleolithic foods are tasty and pleasing to the eye and palette. Break out a new recipe or two that contain strong herbs and spices. Or, convert a favorite family recipe into a favorite Paleo recipe by excluding grains, legumes, or dairy. Substitute squashes for starch, diced tomatoes for sauces, and strong flavors like lemon in place of salt. If you are a little crafty you can turn any recipe into a Paleo recipe.

Here is an example of a common party dip, guacamole, which usually contains healthy items but with large amounts of salt. The following recipe uses all Paleo-approved fresh food items without the salt or canned items found in most recipes.

Party Guacamole

Guacamole is a party favorite that is quite healthy.

INGREDIENTS | **SERVES 4–6**

4 ripe avocados
2 vine-ripe tomatoes, diced
½ cup diced green onions
1 tablespoon diced jalapeño peppers
2 cloves garlic, diced
Juice of 1 lime
Black pepper, to taste

1. Scoop out the flesh of the avocados and place in a small bowl. Mash the avocado with a fork.

2. Add the tomatoes, onions, jalapeños, and garlic. Mix together.

3. Squeeze on fresh lime juice and mix.

4. Add black pepper to taste.

Paleo Thanksgiving Feast

Holidays that are focused around food do not have to be avoided because of the Paleo lifestyle. The flavors of traditional meals can still be shared with the family that abides by the Paleolithic lifestyle. Traditional turkey, baked vegetables, appetizers, and desserts can be enjoyed on Paleo. It may take a little time to find recipe substitutions, but it can be done quite easily.

When trying to design a family meal, it may help to fill in a table with the traditional dish and the substitutions that best work for that original recipe.

HOLIDAY MENU SUBSTITUTION TABLE	
Traditional Recipe	**Possible Substitutions/Changes**
Roasted turkey	Sage, pepper, oregano for salt and roast carrots, broccoli, turnips inside turkey
Turkey gravy	Diced tomatoes, olive oil, and basil reduction sauce
Mashed potatoes	Mashed sweet potatoes with cinnamon, nutmeg, and allspice
Creamed green beans	Sautéed asparagus and Brussels sprouts in flax oil
Rolls and butter	Side salad with oil and lemon/ginger dressing with thyme
Apple pie	Baked whole apples with cinnamon and coconut flakes

It is not difficult to design a scrumptious holiday Paleo meal that the entire family will love. The trick is to find good substitutions that do not make the family think they are missing out on the sugar, high-fructose corn syrup, and bellyache post meal.

Holidays

Holidays are traditional eating events for families and this does not need to change because a family chooses to follow a Paleolithic lifestyle. There are plenty of wholesome, delicious choices that are sure to please everyone. The following menu is sure to appeal to your party guests:

Rosemary Rack of Lamb in Berries Sauce

This rack of lamb recipe is sure to be a winner at any holiday or dinner party. The flavors are strong and the presentation a winner. Your guests won't know it's Paleo.

INGREDIENTS | **SERVES 4**

1 rack of grass-fed lamb, on the bone
Ground black pepper, to taste
2 cloves of crushed garlic, separated
Dried thyme, to taste
2 sprigs of fresh rosemary
2 tablespoons olive oil
1 cup of mixed berries of your choice
1 cup no-salt-added organic beef stock

1. On the rack of lamb, sprinkle black pepper, 1 clove crushed garlic, thyme, and 1 sprig of fresh rosemary.

2. Place lamb in a 400°F oven. Roast for 13 minutes per pound or until internal temperature reaches 135°F. Remove from oven and set aside to rest.

3. Prepare sauce by combining remaining garlic, rosemary, olive oil, berries, and beef stock in a medium pan over low heat. Stir and cook for about 5 minutes.

4. Reduce sauce until thick (may take another 5 minutes) and pour over cooked lamb.

Sautéed Asparagus

Asparagus makes a healthy and filling side complement to any main course. Try this dish with any meat, poultry, or fish recipe.

INGREDIENTS | **SERVES 4**

1 bunch fresh asparagus
2 tablespoons walnut oil
2 cloves chopped garlic

1. Cut bottoms off asparagus, then cut remainder of stalks into 2" pieces.

2. Add walnut oil to a skillet set on medium heat.

3. Add garlic and cook for about 30 seconds, then add asparagus.

4. Stir-fry until asparagus is tender when pierced with fork, approximately 5–8 minutes.

Paleo Brownies

These brownies are quite a treat for the chocolate lover in you. Children and adults both love this recipe.

INGREDIENTS | **YIELDS 9 LARGE OR 16 SMALL BROWNIES**

6 tablespoons oil of your choice

½ cup raw honey

2 eggs

½ cup cacao powder

½ cup cacao nibs

½ cup almond, pecan, or flaxseed meal

¼ cup arrowroot

1. In a large bowl, combine all the ingredients and mix until smooth.

2. Pour contents into greased 8" square baking pan.

3. Bake at 350°F for 20 minutes or until toothpick inserted into the center comes out clean.

Parties and get-togethers are an opportune time to share your new Paleolithic lifestyle with friends and family. Impress them with your delicious recipes then tell them how healthy the food is. How can anyone deny food that tastes great and has lifelong health benefits? The Paleolithic lifestyle will bring you and your guests a lifetime of happiness.

CHAPTER 5

Menu Planning

The secret of success to the Paleolithic lifestyle is in the planning. If you can get into a routine of planning your shopping and meals in advance, eating this way is easy. In fact, you might find it easier than your current lifestyle. Beginning to look at grocery shopping as a pleasure and not a chore will help with a smooth and enjoyable transition.

Implementing the Diet

The first step to implementing the Paleo lifestyle is to figure out what you and your family are going to eat. Using the lists in the appendixes and the general rule that if it was hunted or gathered you can eat it, start to imagine the types of dishes you will make and where and when you are going to prepare them. If you have a busy lifestyle, and working during the day is the norm, preparation in bulk will be your best friend. On the weekends, or every couple of days, cook up a few of your favorite meals and pack them in smaller containers for the refrigerator or freezer. Preparation in advance will make things easy and will reduce the temptation to veer off course.

QUESTION

What do I do if I am out and without a prepared meal?
Eating out Paleo is easier than you might think. Any grilled meat with steamed vegetables or mixed green salad with grilled steak, chicken, or shrimp on top is a perfect Paleo meal. Make sure to ask for lemon and olive oil on the side for a quick, refreshing dressing alternative to balsalmic vinegar.

Let's Go Shopping!

Food shopping can be a tedious task, but when you switch over to Paleo, a plethora of fresh and vibrant color awaits you at the supermarket. Take this opportunity to find excitement in the new fruits, vegetables, meats, and spices at your disposal. If you have never shopped at an organic supermarket like Whole Foods, you will surely delight in the freshness of the selections there. Walk around the aisles and touch and smell all the produce you can get your hands on. Items that you have a positive response to, put in your basket. Don't be afraid to try exotic items you have never thought of eating before such as mustard greens, bok choy, star fruit, and the various squashes on the market today. Lists may be a great way to organize your shopping trip to ensure you get everything you need for the various recipes you will be cooking. Try the following type of list to ensure that foods from all food groups are covered:

Protein	Vegetable	Fruit	Fat
ground beef	broccoli	apples	flax oil
chicken breast	asparagus	strawberries	sunflower seeds
wild salmon	red pepper	blueberries	avocado
haddock	carrots	grapefruit	almond butter
eggs	romaine lettuce	kiwi	olive oil

Organic Versus Non-Organic Foods

In today's agricultural farming, mass production is the name of the game. What can a farm do to get more, more, more produce off of the land with as little loss as possible due to illness or infestation? What that means for the consumer is that you are unknowingly subjected to hormones and harsh chemicals in the form of pesticides and fertilizers used on crops and animals before it enters the grocery store. The land is overused and the food produced has fewer vitamins than the food of our ancestors.

Benefits of Organic Foods

Are organic food items better for you? There are certain facts that cannot be denied.

- Organic produce is not exposed to synthetic pesticides.
- Organic farms use organic fertilizer from farm animals to put nutrients back into the soil.
- Organic food is regulated by national and international government agencies.

Food that is grown by conventional farming is laden with chemicals. These chemicals are poisonous for an unsuspecting insect or other animal, yet are supposedly suitable for human consumption. What amount of these toxins will it take to cause deleterious effects in humans?

Grass-Fed and Free-Range Products

Why should it really matter what the animal product you are eating ate before it got to your plate? The answer to this is more important than you know. Each cell in a living organism is surrounded by a cell membrane. That cell membrane is made up of fatty acids. These fatty acids, omega-3 and omega-6, are considered to be essential because they cannot be produced by the body and must be found in the diet. Living organisms that contain fatty acids have varying ratios of omega-6 to omega-3. The ratio found in healthy humans was found to be less than 4:1. Scientific research has found that the omega ratio profile in grain-fed animals can be as high as 20:1 versus grass-fed animals at around 3:1.

QUESTION

Does grass-fed really make a difference?
According to Jo Robinson, *New York Times* investigative journalist and bestselling author, compared with feedlot meat, meat from grass-fed beef, bison, lambs, and goats has less total fat, saturated fat, cholesterol, and calories. It also has more vitamin E, beta-carotene, vitamin C, and a number of health-promoting fats, including omega-3 fatty acids and "conjugated linoleic acid," or CLA.

Paleo Meal Planning

The road to success with the Paleolithic lifestyle is all in the planning. If you plan your meals well and have plenty of food on hand you will surely be successful. The following steps will help to ensure that you are considering all of the major food groups and portioning your meals to have all macronutrients represented in the plan.

Planning Out the Protein

If you refer back to Chapter 3, you will see the standard formulas for determining your best macronutrient amounts based on your exertion levels. Once you determine your level of activity and lean body mass you can find an amount of protein to feed yourself. This is the first macronutrient to consider in menu planning. Let's use the example from Chapter 3 as a model. A 140-pound woman with 20 percent body fat who exercises lightly (1 to 3 times per week) would need approximately 616 calories of her total for the day to come from protein sources. If this woman decides that she wants to eat five meals a day, then the amount of protein calories per meal comes to 123 calories. There are roughly 4 calories of protein in each gram of protein which equates to 30 grams of protein per meal. That means that she should design her menu to include 30 grams of protein at every meal. The following are some great choices that contain the correct amount of protein for this example:

GOOD PROTEIN SOURCES

Protein Source	Ounces	Grams
Egg white	6	27
Mackerel	4	27
Haddock	4	28
Chicken breast	4	28
Crab meat (real)	5	28
Grouper	4	28
Ground beef	5	29
Swordfish	4	29
Flank steak	4	29
Scallops	6	29
Snapper	5	29

Planning Out the Fat

The average woman has fat gram needs around 40 grams per day, while the average male needs are in the 50 grams per day range. These figures are a starting point. It is not set in stone for every person. Once you have been doing the Paleo lifestyle for a while, you can adjust as needed. If you seem famished often, you may benefit from an increase in good fats. If you feel full all the time, your body may benefit from lowering this level. This is the macronutrient that you can play with a little, unlike protein.

GOOD FAT SOURCES		
Fat	Serving Size	Grams of Fat
Flax oil	1 tablespoon	14
Uddo's oil	1 tablespoon	14
Avocado	½ avocado	14.5
Salmon	3 ounces	22
Black walnuts	3 tablespoons	15
Sesame seeds	4 tablespoons	16

ALERT

Many women tend to gain weight when eating large quantities of nuts and seeds. Women particularly need to be aware that if their desire is to increase their fat content during the day, other sources higher in omega-3 fatty acids, such as flax oil, Uddo's oil, salmon, or avocado are better for optimal health while maintaining a lower body fat percentage.

Planning Out the Carbohydrates

Your carbohydrate consumption will likely be the most challenging change when starting the Paleolithic lifestyle due to the lack of grains, starches, and legumes in the plan. Although it may take time to transition, this is the category with the most selection and diversity. Try to think of this category as a way to have fun with your menu. You can try new and interesting fruits and vegetables that will add color and life to your plate. The total amount of calories left over after determining protein and fat will come from the carbohydrate category, so once you figure out the amount of calories needed, divide by the number of meals and you are on your way. To continue with the current example, the 140-pound woman has 784 calories left over. That will leave her roughly 150 calories each meal to come from carbohydrates.

Developing Meals

Once you have your protein, fat, and carbohydrate portions determined, you can now begin to plan your daily meals. Below is a table with a sample menu:

SAMPLE 1-DAY MENU PLAN			
Meal	**Protein**	**Fat**	**Carbohydrate**
1	6 egg whites		1 cup asparagus and 1 cup tomatoes
2	4 ounces lean turkey	4 tablespoons sesame seeds	1 apple
3	4 ounces chicken breast	1 tablespoon flax oil and lemon juice	3 cups salad
4	3 ounces salmon		2 cups steamed broccoli and ½ grapefruit
5 (post-workout meal)	protein shake		4 ounces sweet potato

Notice that in the menu above there is not a fat at every single meal. This is because you must consider the fat in other parts of the menu. In meal 4 the protein source, salmon, is also a good source of omega-3 fatty acid. That fat must be considered in the total fat for the day.

Cooking and Flavoring Meals

A very important component of any meal plan is the consistency. In order to be consistent you must find a way to escape boredom. If you ask anyone who has ever been on a traditional diet, even those who have been successful on one, they will often complain that they are eating the same foods meal after meal, day after day. That's where cooking and flavoring foods becomes an important component. Experimenting with recipes and trying new foods will keep your plan exciting and fresh instead of mundane and boring.

Preparation of Protein

There are three main ways to cook and prepare food: air heated, moist heated, and microwaving. Each of the three ways of preparation cook food in various amounts of time and certain foods cook better under different conditions. Roasting and broiling foods are examples of air heat cooking and are good methods for steak, chicken, most seafood, lamb, and veal. These meats can stand higher temperatures and cook in shorter amounts of time. Braising and pot roasting of foods are usually done on meats that are not as lean and require longer cooking at lower temperatures. They are often cooked with sauces or in broths to help retain moisture. Examples of meats that would benefit from this style of preparation are pot roasts, pork loin and shanks, whole turkeys, beef chuck, and beef flank.

Alternatives for the Experienced Chef

Once you have your chef's hat on for awhile, you might want to try some other more sophisticated ways to cook. High-heat options are good for quick cooking. They are best for thinner cuts or for meats that do not need to be fully cooked, such as high-end, sushi-grade seafood. Searing food is an indirect high heat method that is done on the top of the stove, preferably over a gas flame. It will cook the outside of meat to add a little flavor and sear in the juice on the inside. This is ideal for tuna steak and high-quality cuts of beef. Broiling in the oven is a method of direct heat with a flame. It brings the flavor of outdoor grilling to the indoor kitchen. Pork and veal chops work well with this type of cooking and quick grilling of seafood can be accomplished this way. Sautéing meats is a medium to medium-high heat method that is great for cooking foods that have smaller surface areas. It is quick, convenient, and does not take much experience to prepare delicious Paleo-friendly meals for the entire family.

Vegetable Preparation

Vegetables are best when eaten raw as they retain their full vitamin and mineral profile. When they must be cooked there are several methods that will produce different tastes and textures. Steaming vegetables is the next best way to eat them next to raw. It is also an easy way to prepare vegetables in bulk to be used over several meals. Just as with meat, sautéing vegetables in oil is a great way to prepare your food. Be aware, however, that you must account for the fat used in cooking the food into your daily fat allowance. Additionally, you must keep in mind that not all oils behave the same way when exposed to heat. When choosing an oil to cook with, you want to consider its viscosity, the way it keeps the food from sticking to itself, and its smoke value (the amount of smoke it produces when it's burned). If an oil produces a great deal of smoke when heated, it will burn off of the food and not provide much for actual cooking.

ALERT

Flax oil is best used in its natural state. When flax is exposed to high heat it can increase the risk of releasing free radicals, which has been linked to diseases such as cancer.

Obtaining Fat in Your Diet

There are several ways to include good fats into your diet. You can add it directly onto your food so it is eaten in its natural state. It can be mixed with other items to make a great salad dressing or marinade. As stated previously, it can be used while sautéing foods. Fats used to cook with produce different results and flavors and are nice additives to a recipe. Olive oil is a viscose and great-tasting oil for cooking. Coconut oil is nice to add a crispy effect to food. Walnut and grapeseed oils are best for low temperature heating and for use in dessert or marinade recipes. Sesame oil is a great additive at the very end of cooking for a bit of flavor.

Bring on the Flavor

Spices are dried seasonings that come from the bark, buds, fruit, roots, or seeds of plants while herbs are from the leaves. Herbs are fresh and have a short shelf life, a week or less. Spices will generally last up to six months in a cool, dark storage area. Spices and fresh herbs should become a mainstay for the Paleolithic eater. There are a plethora of different fresh and dried spices from around the world that can be used to liven up any dish or recipe. As a Paleo eater, you need to avoid cooking and eating the same things time and time again. This is the absolute worst trap for a Paleolithic cook to fall into. Preparing every meal the same way will not only become boring, but all of your food will start to taste the same, thus causing you to dislike the plan. Spices and a variety of cooking styles will ensure that you engage many of your taste buds in your meals and keep your interest high. Below are examples of good spices and herbs to try and their accompanying food items best used for:

SPICES	
Spice/Herb	Best Use
Basil	Tomato
Cilantro	Salsa, salad dressing, tuna
Cinnamon	Carrot, sweet potato
Clove	Pork
Curry	Meats, poultry, soups, eggs
Lemon	Steamed vegetables, fish, poultry
Mustard seed	Meat, fish, poultry, salad dressing
Onion	All dishes
Oregano	Salads, sauces
Rosemary	Lamb, chicken, fish
Sage	Pork, veal, tomato sauces
Tarragon	Meat, poultry, fish
Thyme	Slow cooked meals, slow cooker meats

FACT

Spices from around the world are used to maintain freshness of food. You'll notice that warmer climates tend to have "spicier" food. This is because food spoilage is more of an issue in warmer climates. Additionally, some spices have antibacterial properties to promote better health.

Although this list above is helpful to start, the best way to learn to use spices and herbs is to experiment. Open and smell every spice you can get your hands on and throw the spices that pique your interest into your dishes. A good rule is to use fresh, leafy herbs toward the end of your cooking, but also in the beginning of recipes that are uncooked to absorb flavor such as cilantro in guacamole. Spices are usually used at the beginning of recipes so that their flavors will be well established in the dishes such as sage and thyme added to a roasted chicken.

CHAPTER 6

Tasty Breakfasts

Mini Quiche

These are a tasty treat for breakfast or anytime and can be made in bulk.

INGREDIENTS | SERVES 8

6 large eggs
6 slices nitrate-free bacon
Cooking spray
½ cup broccoli, chopped
½ cup mushrooms, sliced
½ cup onions, diced
½ cup red peppers, diced

1. Preheat oven to 325°F. Line muffin tin with 8 foil cups.

2. Whisk 6 eggs and set aside.

3. Cook bacon until crisp, drain on paper towels, and chop into ½" pieces.

4. Spray a medium sauté pan with cooking spray. Sauté all remaining ingredients for 5 minutes.

5. Pour eggs into foil cups, filling each ⅔ of the way.

6. Add bacon and vegetables to each cup.

7. Bake 25 minutes or until golden brown.

PER SERVING Calories: 118 | Fat: 8.5 g | Protein: 8 g | Sodium: 198 mg | Fiber: 0.5 g | Carbohydrate: 2 g

Breakfast Salad

Salad isn't just for lunch and dinner anymore. When you are on the Paleolithic diet plan, salads are round-the-clock meals.

INGREDIENTS | SERVES 1

3 cups baby spinach leaves

4 large eggs, hard-boiled, peeled, and quartered

2 slices nitrate-free bacon, cooked and chopped

½ cup cucumber, sliced

½ avocado, diced

½ apple, sliced

Juice of ½ lemon

1. Arrange spinach leaves on a plate and top with eggs and bacon.

2. Add cucumber, avocado, and apple slices to top of salad.

3. Squeeze fresh lemon juice over the salad. Serve immediately.

PER SERVING Calories: 694 | Fat: 44 g | Protein: 40 g | Sodium: 1,013 mg | Fiber: 10 g | Carbohydrate: 31 g

Bacon and Vegetable Omelet

Bacon and eggs are a breakfast tradition and they are 100 percent Paleo-approved.

INGREDIENTS | SERVES 2

6 slices nitrate-free bacon, diced

1 yellow summer squash, chopped

1 cup mushrooms, sliced

1 zucchini, chopped

¼ cup fresh basil leaves, diced

2 tablespoons olive oil

8 large eggs, beaten

1. In a large sauté pan, cook bacon until crispy. Add the vegetables and basil to the pan and sauté until tender, approximately 5–8 minutes.

2. Heat olive oil in a second sauté pan over medium heat.

3. Cook eggs for 3 minutes on each side.

4. Place the vegetable and bacon mixture on one half of the eggs and fold over the other half to enclose the filling. Serve.

PER SERVING Calories: 670 | Fat: 52 g | Protein: 39 g | Sodium: 849 mg | Fiber: 2 g | Carbohydrate: 11 g

Easy Pancake Recipe

This pancake recipe is quick and easy and can be multiplied to make enough for an entire family. Once cooked, sprinkle the pancake with cinnamon or a small amount of agave nectar for an old-fashioned pancake taste.

INGREDIENTS | SERVES 1

1 banana
1 large egg
1 teaspoon nut butter of choice
2 teaspoons coconut oil

Bananas as Thickeners

Bananas can be a good replacement for flour. Bananas act as thickening agents in recipes that would normally be too fluid.

1. In a small bowl, mash banana with a fork.

2. Beat egg and add to banana.

3. Add nut butter and mix well.

4. Lightly coat frying pan or griddle with oil and pour entire pancake mixture onto preheated pan.

5. Cook until lightly brown on each side, about 2 minutes per side.

PER SERVING Calories: 389 | Fat: 17 g | Protein: 9.5 g | Sodium: 66 mg | Fiber: 7 g | Carbohydrate: 54 g

Egg Muffins

These are great to make in advance and take on the go.
They are also quite tasty with some sliced avocado.

INGREDIENTS | SERVES 18

2 tablespoons olive oil
12 large eggs
2 medium zucchini
1 bell pepper
1 green onion (optional)
3 cups fresh spinach
1 cup cooked ham

1. Preheat oven to 350°F.

2. Grease two muffin pans with olive oil.

3. In a large bowl, whisk eggs well.

4. In a food processor, process zucchini, pepper, and green onion (if using) until finely chopped, but not smooth.

5. Add chopped vegetables to the eggs.

6. Finely chop spinach in the food processor and add to the egg mixture.

7. Stir in the ham and mix well.

8. Fill the muffin pans halfway with the egg mixture.

9. Bake for 20–25 minutes or until the eggs are set in the middle.

PER SERVING Calories: 75 | Fat: 5 g | Protein: 5 g | Sodium: 108 mg | Fiber: 0.5 g | Carbohydrate: 2 g

Banana-Coconut Bread

This banana-coconut loaf recipe can double as a dessert recipe quite nicely. Serve with fresh banana and strawberry slices for a completely yummy treat.

INGREDIENTS | SERVES 8

1¼ cups almond meal
2 teaspoons baking powder
¼ teaspoon baking soda
½ cup fruit purée
¼ teaspoon cinnamon
2 large eggs
3 large ripe bananas, mashed
¼ cup flaxseed flour
½ cup chopped walnuts
1 cup unsweetened coconut flakes

Fruit Pureés

Fruit purées are a great way to add sweetness to any recipe. Simply place your favorite fruits into a food processor and quickly pulse to chop finely. Use in place of syrups and jams.

1. Preheat oven to 350°F. Grease a loaf pan.

2. Combine the almond meal, baking powder, baking soda, fruit purée, cinnamon, eggs, bananas, and flaxseed flour in a large bowl. Mix well.

3. Fold chopped walnuts and coconut flakes into the batter (do not over-mix). Pour batter into prepared pan.

4. Bake for about 45 minutes or until wooden toothpick comes out dry.

5. Let the bread sit for 5 minutes then transfer to a wire rack and cool completely.

PER SERVING Calories: 264 | Fat: 12 g | Protein: 5.5 g | Sodium: 26 mg | Fiber: 6 g | Carbohydrate: 38 g

Protein Smoothie

This protein shake is a nutritious way to have a good meal on the go. You don't need to leave the house without breakfast anymore when you can make this fast, take-away breakfast.

INGREDIENTS | SERVES 1

1 scoop of vanilla flavor whey or egg protein powder

8 ounces no-sugar-added coconut water

1 tablespoon almond butter

Dash cinnamon

Dash nutmeg

Add all the ingredients to a blender, mix, and enjoy.

PER SERVING Calories: 194 | Fat: 10 g | Protein: 16 g | Sodium: 417 mg | Fiber: 3 g | Carbohydrate: 13 g

Protein Shakes

Protein shakes are the perfect way to give your body what it needs after exercise or a race event. They are quick and transportable, and they taste great!

Strawberry-Banana Pancake

These pancakes are a great alternative to an egg, which tends to be the go-to Paleolithic diet breakfast choice.

INGREDIENTS | SERVES 1

Cooking spray
3 egg whites, lightly beaten
1 banana, sliced
3–4 strawberries, sliced
1 tablespoon almond butter
½ teaspoon cinnamon

1. Preheat a small frying pan coated with cooking spray.

2. Combine egg whites, banana, strawberries, and almond butter in a medium bowl and mix well.

3. Pour into pan, cover with lid, and cook, about 2–3 minutes.

4. Flip pancake to brown the other side.

5. Serve warm with cinnamon sprinkled on top.

PER SERVING Calories: 279 | Fat: 10 g | Protein: 19 g | Sodium: 195 mg | Fiber: 5 g | Carbohydrate: 34 g

Antioxidant Fruit and Nut Salad

Fruit salad can be eaten any time of day, but is particularly good for breakfast. Berries are packed full of antioxidants and walnuts have one of the best omega profiles for nuts to reduce inflammation. This is a winning combination.

INGREDIENTS | SERVES 2

½ cup strawberries, sliced

½ cup raspberries

½ cup blackberries

½ cup blueberries

½ cup mulberries, dried

½ cup chopped walnuts

Combine all ingredients and enjoy.

PER SERVING Calories: 282 | Fat: 20 g | Protein: 6.5 g | Sodium: 5.5 mg | Fiber: 8.5 g | Carbohydrate: 24 g

Poached Eggs

Poached eggs are very quick to make, but you must watch them or they will overcook. Time them exactly to get a perfect poached egg every time.

INGREDIENTS | **SERVES 1**

Water

2 large eggs

1 teaspoon apple cider vinegar

Vinegar on Paleo

Strict Paleolithic dieters do not use vinegar because it was not available during the Paleolithic time period. If you are less strict, you can use it in salad dressings and in cooking. If you use it, try to limit the intake to no more than a couple times a week to promote good pH levels in your body.

1. Bring water to boil in a medium saucepan. Reduce heat to medium-low so that the water is simmering.

2. Add apple cider vinegar to water.

3. Crack and carefully slide eggs into the water.

4. Cook for exactly 3 minutes, remove with a slotted spoon, and serve.

PER SERVING Calories: 150 | Fat: 10 g | Protein: 12 g | Sodium: 126 mg | Fiber: 0 g | Carbohydrate: 2 g

Salmon Omelet

This omelet is full of omega-3 fatty acids. It is well-seasoned and will surely become a breakfast staple.

INGREDIENTS | **SERVES 2**

2 tablespoons olive oil
¼ cup green onions, chopped
1 cup asparagus, trimmed and chopped
1 tablespoon chopped fresh dill
6 ounces salmon
6 large eggs, beaten

1. In a large skillet, combine olive oil, green onions, asparagus, and fresh dill. Sauté until asparagus is soft, 5–10 minutes, and set aside.

2. In same skillet sauté salmon until flaky, about 10 minutes depending on thickness of steak. Set aside.

3. Wipe out the skillet and cook eggs on both sides until lightly browned, about 5 minutes each side.

4. Place salmon and asparagus mixture on half of egg, fold over, and serve.

PER SERVING Calories: 490 | Fat: 33 g | Protein: 40 g | Sodium: 332 mg | Fiber: 4 g | Carbohydrate: 9 g

Paleo Breakfast Bowl

This breakfast is a bit more exciting than the ordinary breakfast you might be used to. Nitrate-free, uncured bacon is a real treat.

INGREDIENTS | SERVES 1

2 tablespoons olive oil
½ cup uncured bacon, diced
1 cup asparagus, diced
2 large eggs

1. Heat olive oil in skillet over medium-high heat.

2. Cook bacon and asparagus in skillet until asparagus is not quite tender. About 8–10 minutes. Remove to small bowl.

3. In the same skillet, cook eggs over easy (do not flip) about 5 minutes. Be sure that yolks are runny.

4. Place cooked eggs on top of bacon mixture.

5. Mix and serve.

PER SERVING Calories: 559 | Fat: 49 g | Protein: 23 g | Sodium: 534 mg | Fiber: 3 g | Carbohydrate: 7.5 g

CHAPTER 7

Luscious Lunchtime

Easy Slow Cooker Pork Tenderloin

Slow cooker meals are a great way to cook for your family. Large quantities can be thrown into the cooker hours in advance. Most leftovers can be easily frozen for future meals.

INGREDIENTS | SERVES 4

1 pound lean pork loin, whole

1 (28-ounce) can diced tomatoes, no salt added

3 medium zucchinis, diced

4 cups cauliflower florets

Chopped fresh basil, to taste

Garlic, to taste

1. Combine all ingredients in a slow cooker.

2. Cook on low for 6–7 hours.

PER SERVING Calories: 165 | Fat: 6.5 g | Protein: 19 g | Sodium: 336 mg | Fiber: 4 g | Carbohydrate: 9.6 g

Low-Fat Meat Choice

Pork is a nice low-fat protein source. It is versatile for cooking and quite flavorful. This often-overlooked meat is a fantastic friend of the Paleolithic lifestyle.

Paleo Pulled Pork

This pulled pork recipe has super flavors. Adjust the spices as needed to kick it up a notch or cool it down. Either way, this recipe is sure to please the entire family.

INGREDIENTS | SERVES 8

2½ pounds pork loin

1 large onion, chopped

1 (16-ounce) can unsalted organic tomato paste

3 tablespoons olive oil

2 cups lemon juice

½ cup unsalted beef broth

4 cloves garlic

¼ teaspoon cayenne pepper

½ teaspoon paprika

2 teaspoons chipotle chili powder

1 teaspoon thyme

1 teaspoon cumin

1. Combine all ingredients in a slow cooker.

2. Cook on low for 5 hours or until meat is softened completely.

3. Once cooled, shred with fork and serve.

PER SERVING Calories: 382 | Fat: 17 g | Protein: 40 g | Sodium: 138 mg | Fiber: 3.5 g | Carbohydrate: 18 g

Chicken Stew with Meat Sauce

This easy-to-make chicken stew is sure to please the entire family. Both kids and adults love this delicious recipe. Serve alone or pour over spaghetti squash as a bolognaise-type sauce.

INGREDIENTS | SERVES 4

1 pound (90 percent lean) grass-fed ground beef

4 boneless, skinless chicken breasts

1 (6-ounce) can organic tomato paste

1 (28-ounce) can diced organic tomatoes, no salt added

4 garlic cloves, chopped

4 large carrots, sliced

2 red bell peppers, diced

2 green bell peppers, diced

1 tablespoon dried thyme

2 tablespoons olive oil

1 tablespoon chili powder

1. In a medium sauté pan, cook ground beef until browned, about 5 minutes. Drain and place in slow cooker.

2. Wipe out pan and place over medium-high heat. Brown the chicken breasts (5 minutes per side). Add to slow cooker.

3. Combine all remaining ingredients in slow cooker.

4. Cook on high for 5 hours.

5. Serve over your favorite steamed vegetable.

PER SERVING Calories: 605 | Fat: 18 g | Protein: 74 g | Sodium: 666 mg | Fiber: 10 g | Carbohydrate: 42 g

Slow Cookers Are Lifesavers

Slow cookers are the greatest appliance for the Paleo enthusiast. These little counter-top cookers allow you to cook easily and in bulk, which is important for a successful Paleolithic dieter.

Stuffed Tomatoes

A vegetarian lunch option that is packed with flavor.

INGREDIENTS	SERVES 3

3 large beefsteak tomatoes
6 small button mushrooms, sliced
4 cloves garlic, minced
6 pieces sun-dried tomatoes, chopped
1 teaspoon ground black pepper
½ teaspoon paprika
1 teaspoon thyme
8 leaves fresh basil, torn

1. Preheat oven to 350°F.

2. Hollow out the tomatoes, reserving tomato pulp. Place tomatoes in a small baking dish.

3. Mix tomato pulp with mushrooms, garlic, sun-dried tomatoes, pepper, paprika, thyme, and basil.

4. Fill tomatoes with tomato pulp mixture and bake for 25 minutes.

PER SERVING Calories: 116 | Fat: 2.5 | Protein: 7.5 g | Sodium: 162 mg | Fiber: 5.5 g | Carbohydrate: 23 g

Chicken Piccata

Chicken is a staple for the Paleolithic eater. This lunchtime treat is a pleasant departure from the ordinary.

INGREDIENTS | SERVES 4

1 cup no-salt-added chicken broth

½ cup lemon juice

4 skinless, boneless chicken breasts

3 tablespoons olive oil

1 cup chopped onion

1 garlic clove, minced

2 cups chopped artichoke hearts

3 tablespoons capers

1 teaspoon pepper

Capers

Capers are salted and should be used only occasionally for a dish such as this one where they are an integral ingredient for a recipe favorite. This dish is still full of flavor without them and will be a delightful treat for your family.

1. Combine chicken broth, lemon juice, and chicken in shallow dish. Cover and marinate overnight in the refrigerator.

2. Heat olive oil in a medium sauté pan and cook onion and garlic until softened, about 2 minutes.

3. Remove chicken from marinade, reserving marinade. Add chicken to pan and brown each side, 5–10 minutes.

4. Add artichoke hearts, capers, pepper, and reserved marinade. Reduce heat and simmer until chicken is thoroughly cooked, another 10 minutes approximately.

PER SERVING Calories: 269 | Fat: 13 g | Protein: 35 g | Sodium: 390 mg | Fiber: 1 g | Carbohydrate: 5 g

Tuna Salad with a Kick

Tuna is a great lunch or snack. It is naturally low in fat, low in calories, and quite flavorful.

INGREDIENTS | 3 SERVINGS

2 (7-ounce) cans chunk light tuna in water

20 green olives, chopped

½ cup green onions, chopped

3 tablespoons capers

1 jalapeño pepper, finely chopped

1 red bell pepper, chopped

2 tablespoons olive oil

2 tablespoons red chili flakes

Juice of 3 lemons

1. Mix all ingredients in a large bowl.

2. Serve chilled alone or over lettuce greens.

PER SERVING Calories: 267 | Fat: 15 g | Protein: 30 g | Sodium: 1,072 mg | Fiber: 2 g | Carbohydrate: 4.5 g

Quick Meals

Organic, no-salt-added tuna is a staple in the Paleolithic chef's kitchen. You can whip up a quick lunch or dinner on a moment's notice and you'll get plenty of low-fat protein.

Shredded Chicken Wraps

Wraps are a great way to get the feel of a tortilla wrap without the forbidden carbohydrates. You can easily substitute your favorite meat or fish for the chicken to vary your lunchtime menu.

INGREDIENTS | **SERVES 8**

2 boneless, skinless chicken breasts (baked, poached, or broiled)

2 celery stalks, chopped

¼ cup chopped basil

2 tablespoons olive oil

2 tablespoons lemon juice

1 teaspoon minced garlic

Ground black pepper, to taste

1 head of radicchio or romaine lettuce

1. Shred or finely chop chicken and place in a medium bowl.

2. Mix chicken with celery, basil, olive oil, lemon juice, garlic, and pepper.

3. Separate lettuce leaves and place on 8 plates.

4. Spoon chicken mixture onto lettuce leaves and roll up.

PER SERVING Calories: 123 | Fat: 3.5 g | Protein: 9 g | Sodium: 14 mg | Fiber: 0.5 g | Carbohydrate: 1 g

Roasted Pork Tenderloin

When you have a bit more time and want to prepare for a large family gathering, this is the recipe to go for. It serves ten easily and will wow your guests with its flavorful punch.

INGREDIENTS | SERVES 10

2½ pounds pork loin
Juice of 1 large orange
3 tablespoons lime juice
2 tablespoons red wine
10 cloves of garlic, minced
2 tablespoons dried rosemary
1 tablespoon ground black pepper

1. Combine all ingredients in a shallow dish or large zip-top plastic bag. Refrigerate and marinate pork for at least 2 hours.

2. Remove pork from marinade and bring to room temperature. Preheat oven to 350°F.

3. Cook for 20–25 minutes, or until the internal temperature reaches 165°F. Allow the pork to rest for 5 minutes before carving.

PER SERVING Calories: 218 | Fat: 9.5 g | Protein: 30 g | Sodium: 53 mg | Fiber: 0 g | Carbohydrate: 1 g

Chicken Enchiladas

If you have been craving a Mexican feast, try this spicy Paleolithic alternative. This recipe has most of the taste of traditional enchiladas without the carbohydrates.

INGREDIENTS | SERVES 8

2 tablespoons olive oil

2 pounds boneless, skinless chicken breast, cut in 1" cubes

4 cloves garlic, minced

½ cup onion, finely chopped

2 cups chopped tomatoes

1 teaspoon ground cumin

1 teaspoon chili powder

½ cup fresh cilantro

Juice from 2 limes

1 (10-ounce) package frozen chopped spinach, thawed and drained

8 collard green leaves

1. Heat olive oil in a medium skillet. Sauté chicken, garlic, and onion in the hot oil until thoroughly cooked, about 10 minutes.

2. Add tomatoes, cumin, chili powder, cilantro, and lime juice and simmer for 5 minutes.

3. Add spinach and simmer for 5 more minutes. Remove from heat.

4. In a separate pan, quickly steam collard greens to soften, about 3 minutes.

5. Wrap chicken mixture in collard greens and serve.

PER SERVING Calories: 141 | Fat: 5 g | Protein: 22 g | Sodium: 35 mg | Fiber: 2 g | Carbohydrate: 5 g

Curried Chicken Salad

The recipe makes two servings, but you can double or triple the amounts.
You can also change the spices around for more variety.

INGREDIENTS | SERVES 2

2 tablespoons olive oil

8 ounces chicken breast, cubed

1 stalk celery, sliced

1 small onion, diced

½ English cucumber, diced

½ cup almonds, chopped

2 apples, chopped

½ teaspoon curry powder

4 cups baby romaine lettuce

1. In sauté pan, cook chicken, celery, and onion thoroughly in hot olive oil for 5–10 minutes. Set aside to cool.

2. In mixing bowl combine cucumber, almonds, apples, and curry powder with the cooled chicken mixture.

3. Serve over bed of baby romaine lettuce.

PER SERVING Calories: 431 | Fat: 27 g | Protein: 27 g | Sodium: 31 mg | Fiber: 8 g | Carbohydrate: 28 g

Cage Free

Cage-free, barn-roaming chickens are an important component of the Paleolithic diet. Chickens raised in commercial chicken farms are fed a corn-based diet with low omega-3 fatty acid content. Additionally, they are kept in coops where they get little exercise and are fed antibiotics to maintain their health. All things injected into your meat sources will filter up through your food.

Chicken with Sautéed Tomatoes and Pine Nuts

Sautéed tomatoes and pine nuts add a nice, nutty flavor to an ordinary dish.
This topping can be added to fish or beef just as easily.

INGREDIENTS | **SERVES 2**

¼ cup olive oil
1 cup cherry tomatoes, halved
¼ cup green chilies, chopped
¼ cup cilantro
½ cup pine nuts
2 boneless skinless chicken breasts

1. Heat olive oil in a medium skillet over medium-high heat. Sauté tomatoes, chilies, cilantro, and pine nuts until golden brown, about 5 minutes. Set aside.

2. In the same pan, cook chicken 5 minutes on each side.

3. Return tomato mixture to pan and cover. Simmer on low for 5 minutes until chicken is fully cooked.

PER SERVING Calories: 595 | Fat: 45 g | Protein: 44 g | Sodium: 6.5 mg | Fiber: 2 g | Carbohydrate: 8 g

Zesty Pecan Chicken and Grape Salad

Coating your chicken with nuts adds a crispy skin to keep the breast inside moist and tender.

INGREDIENTS | SERVES 6

¼ cup pecans, chopped

1 teaspoon chili powder

¼ cup olive oil

1½ pounds boneless, skinless chicken breasts

1½ cups white grapes

6 cups salad greens

Toasting Nuts for Fresher Flavor and Crispness

To wake the natural flavor of the nuts, heat them on the stovetop or in the oven for a few minutes. For the stovetop, spread nuts in a dry skillet, and heat over a medium flame until their natural oils come to the surface. For the oven, spread the nuts in a single layer on a baking sheet, and toast for 5 to 10 minutes at 350°F, until the oils are visible. Cool nuts before serving.

1. Preheat oven to 400°F.

2. In a blender, mix the chopped nuts and chili powder. Pour in the oil while the blender is running. When the mixture is thoroughly combined, pour it into a shallow bowl.

3. Coat the chicken with the pecan mixture and place on racked baking dish; roast for 40–50 minutes, until the chicken is thoroughly cooked. Remove from oven, let cool for 5 minutes, and thinly slice.

4. Slice the grapes and tear the greens into bite-size pieces. To serve, fan the chicken over the greens and sprinkle with sliced grapes.

PER SERVING Calories: 220 | Fat: 13 g | Protein: 21 g | Sodium: 11 mg | Fiber: 1 g | Carbohydrate: 5.5 g

Delicious Dinner

Thai Coconut Scallops

These scallops cook in 10 minutes and taste as if you were cooking all day. Great for dinner or for special occasions.

INGREDIENTS | SERVES 4

1 tablespoon olive oil
1 pound large scallops
½ medium onion, chopped
1 (13.5-ounce) can coconut milk
2 tablespoons hot curry powder
1 teaspoon cumin
¼ cup flaked coconut
8–10 leaves fresh basil, slivered

Health Benefits of Scallops

Scallops are rich in omega-3 fatty acids. Additionally, they are a great source of vitamin B_{12}, potassium, magnesium, and selenium, which has been shown to neutralize free radicals in the body.

1. Heat olive oil in a medium skillet over medium-high heat.

2. Sauté scallops and onion in olive oil until browned, 5–8 minutes depending on thickness of scallops.

3. Add coconut milk, curry powder, cumin, and coconut.

4. Bring to a light boil and simmer for 10 minutes.

5. Garnish with basil.

PER SERVING Calories: 409 | Fat: 31 g | Protein: 28 g | Sodium: 317 mg | Fiber: 3 g | Carbohydrate: 7 g

Curried Shrimp with Veggies

This curried shrimp and vegetable dish is quick and easy, but quite authentic-tasting. It is sure to please everyone in your family who is fond of foods from India.

INGREDIENTS | SERVES 4

2 tablespoons olive oil

1 tablespoon green curry powder

1 pound wild Argentinian shrimp, peeled and deveined

1 (12-ounce) bag frozen broccoli florets

4 large carrots, sliced

1 (8-ounce) can coconut milk

1. In a skillet over medium heat, warm olive oil and green curry powder.

2. Add shrimp, broccoli, carrots, and coconut milk.

3. Cook until all vegetables are tender and coconut milk cooks down to a thick, paste-like consistency (approximately 15 minutes).

PER SERVING Calories: 343 | Fat: 21 g | Protein: 22 g | Sodium: 250 mg | Fiber: 6 g | Carbohydrate: 21 g

Turkey Meatballs

This is a fairly generic meatball recipe with some basic additions. You can substitute any type of ground meat you prefer: bison, beef, chicken, or pork. Flaxseed meal can replace the almond meal as well.

INGREDIENTS | SERVES 8

2 pounds (93 percent lean) ground turkey

1 cup almond meal

2 large eggs

5 scallions, chopped

1 red bell pepper, diced

2 cloves garlic, minced

1 tablespoon dried basil

1 tablespoon dried oregano

2 tablespoons olive oil

Higher Fat Ground Meats

Although most people make sure to buy the lowest fat ground meat, it is more beneficial to buy fattier ground meat when it is from grass-fed or barn-roaming animals. This meat is lower in saturated fat than most commercial ground meat, and the fat profiles favor the omega-3 fatty acids to fight inflammation and heart disease in your body.

1. Preheat oven to 400°F.

2. Combine all ingredients except olive oil in a large bowl. Mix well with clean hands.

3. Add olive oil to turkey mixture and mix well.

4. Form turkey mixture into 24 meatballs and place on 2 rimmed baking pans.

5. Bake for 20 minutes.

PER SERVING Calories: 198 | Fat: 6 g | Protein: 29 g | Sodium: 21 mg | Fiber: 1.5 g | Carbohydrate: 13 g

Paleo Spaghetti

*This is a great alternative to traditional pasta. Serve with sauce and turkey meatballs
for a great Paleolithic take on Grandma's spaghetti and meatball recipe!*

INGREDIENTS | SERVES 4

1 large spaghetti squash

Pasta Alternative

Spaghetti squash is a fantastic carbohydrate source for all you pasta addicts out
there. This squash looks like spaghetti
when the meat is peeled from the skin. It
has the relative texture of pasta. And, most
importantly, it is quite filling.

1. Preheat oven to 350°F.

2. Cut squash in half lengthwise.

3. Place cut-side down in baking dish with ¼" water.

4. Cook 30 minutes, then turn over and cook until soft all
   the way through with fork, approximately 10 minutes.

5. Shred with fork and serve.

PER SERVING Calories: 94 | Fat: 0 g | Protein: 2 g |
Sodium: 1.5 mg | Fiber: 0 g | Carbohydrate: 20 g

Grilled Jerk Chicken

This marinated chicken dish is great to cook in large quantities for eating throughout the week. It is a fantastic summer dish to make outside on the grill.

INGREDIENTS | **SERVES 4**

5 cloves chopped garlic
1 teaspoon ginger powder
1 teaspoon dried thyme
1 teaspoon ground paprika
1 teaspoon ground cinnamon
½ teaspoon ground allspice
½ cup lemon juice
½ cup red wine
4 boneless, skinless chicken breasts

1. Combine garlic, ginger, thyme, paprika, cinnamon, allspice, lemon juice, and red wine in a large bowl.

2. Add chicken and marinate for at least 5 hours in refrigerator.

3. Prepare a charcoal or gas grill.

4. Remove chicken from marinade and wrap in aluminum foil. Place foil packets on preheated grill and cook for 12 minutes.

5. Remove chicken from aluminum foil and grill for 5 minutes.

PER SERVING Calories: 161 | Fat: 1.5 g | Protein: 35 g | Sodium: 0.5 mg | Fiber: 0 g | Carbohydrate: 2 g

Pecan-Crusted Chicken

This pecan crust recipe is quite versatile. It works for fish as well as chicken, and other nuts can be substituted for different flavors.

INGREDIENTS | SERVES 4

1 cup finely chopped pecans
2 large eggs, beaten
4 boneless, skinless chicken breasts

1. Preheat oven to 350°F.

2. Place chopped nuts in a shallow bowl and eggs in a separate shallow bowl.

3. Dip each chicken breast in egg and then in nuts. Place coated chicken breasts in a shallow baking dish.

4. Bake for 25 minutes.

PER SERVING Calories: 377 | Fat: 24 g | Protein: 40 g | Sodium: 32 mg | Fiber: 3 g | Carbohydrate: 4 g

Sour Cherry Beef Stew

This recipe was adapted from a traditional non–Paleolithic diet beef stew recipe. You will be surprised at how good this really tastes.

INGREDIENTS | SERVES 10

¼ cup almond flour

½ teaspoon nutmeg

1 teaspoon cinnamon

½ teaspoon allspice

½ teaspoon ground black pepper

2 pounds chuck steak, cubed

2 tablespoons olive oil

2 medium onions, chopped

2 (16-ounce) cans sour cherries (reserve half of the juice)

½ cup red wine

2 pounds button mushrooms, quartered

1 (14-ounce) can organic beef broth, unsalted

½ cup water

Alcohol in Cooking

Alcohol in general is not allowed on the Paleolithic plan, but some chefs find it acceptable to use alcohol while cooking, since most of the alcohol is burned off. This is a nice way to bring some flavor to a dish without worrying about altering the plan significantly.

1. Combine almond flour, nutmeg, cinnamon, allspice, and pepper in a plastic bag.

2. Add chuck steak to plastic bag and shake to coat evenly.

3. Heat olive oil in a large skillet over medium-high heat.

4. Sear steak quickly in skillet for 1–2 minutes each side. Remove from skillet and place in slow cooker.

5. Using the same skillet, cook onion on medium heat for 8 minutes.

6. Add cherries, juice, and red wine to the skillet and cook for 5 more minutes, until the onions are browned.

7. Pour the cherry mixture into slow cooker.

8. Add broth, mushrooms, and water to slow cooker. Cook for at least 5 hours on low heat in slow cooker.

PER SERVING Calories: 307 | Fat: 16 g | Protein: 24 g | Sodium: 197 mg | Fiber: 3 g | Carbohydrate: 16 g

Roasted Pork Tenderloin

This pork tenderloin recipe will melt in your mouth.

INGREDIENTS | SERVES 6

Juice of 1 large orange
3 tablespoons lime juice
2 tablespoons red wine
10 whole cloves of garlic
1 teaspoon dried thyme
Fresh ground black pepper, to taste
2½ pounds pork loin

1. Combine juices, wine, garlic, thyme, and pepper in a large zip-top plastic bag.

2. Add pork to the bag and marinate pork for at least 2 hours in refrigerator.

3. Preheat oven to 350°F. Remove pork from marinade and place in a shallow baking pan.

4. Cook for 30 minutes or until the internal temperature reaches 165°F.

5. Remove from baking pan and let pork sit for 5 minutes before carving.

PER SERVING Calories: 364 | Fat: 16 g | Protein: 50 g | Sodium: 88 mg | Fiber: 1 g | Carbohydrate: 1.5 g

Chipotle-Lime Mashed Sweet Potato

Sweet potatoes are a great post-workout food. These chipotle-lime mashed potatoes will be a favorite at any family table.

INGREDIENTS | SERVES 10

3 pounds sweet potatoes

1½ tablespoons coconut oil

1¼ teaspoons chipotle powder

Juice from ½ large lime

Alternatives to Sweet Potatoes

If you don't like sweet potatoes, you can easily substitute some lower glycemic-load vegetables such as rutabgas, turnips, or beets. Additionally, cauliflower makes a great fake "mashed potato" substitute.

1. Peel the sweet potatoes and cut into cubes.

2. Steam the cubes until soft, approximately 5–8 minutes. Transfer to a large bowl.

3. In a small saucepan, heat coconut oil and whisk in the chipotle powder and lime juice.

4. Pour the mixture into the bowl with the sweet potato cubes and mash with fork or potato masher.

PER SERVING Calories: 135 | Fat: 2 g | Protein: 2.5 g | Sodium: 75 mg | Fiber: 4 g | Carbohydrate: 27 g

Coconut Crumbed Chicken

This is an easy way to add some flavor and crunch to the chicken (it can be easily adapted to use on firm fish and shrimp). It is also a great way for little kids to enjoy eating with their hands.

INGREDIENTS | SERVES 8

1 cup ground almond meal

2 large eggs

2 teaspoons ground pepper

1 tablespoon Italian seasoning

1 cup ground unsweetened coconut flakes

½ cup flaxseed meal

4 tablespoons coconut oil

16 chicken tenderloins

1. Pour almond meal into a shallow bowl. In another bowl, whisk eggs, ground pepper, and Italian seasoning. In a third bowl, combine coconut flakes with flaxseed meal.

2. Coat the chicken pieces with the almond meal.

3. Transfer the chicken to the egg mixture, then coat with the coconut mixture.

4. Heat the coconut oil in a large nonstick skillet over medium-high heat.

5. Pan-fry the tenderloins until cooked through, approximately 5 minutes on each side, depending on thickness of chicken.

PER SERVING Calories: 323 | Fat: 19 g | Protein: 37 g | Sodium: 21 mg | Fiber: 2 g | Carbohydrate: 4 g

Steamed King Crab Legs

Shellfish is a healthy and flavorful protein source. It is naturally low in fat and has a nice, sweet taste. A great alternative to the usual poultry or beef dish.

INGREDIENTS	SERVES 4

2 tablespoons oil
3 cloves garlic, crushed
1 (1") piece fresh gingerroot, crushed
1 stalk lemongrass, crushed
2 pounds Alaskan king crab legs
1 teaspoon ground black pepper

1. Heat the oil in a large pot over medium-high heat.

2. Add the garlic, ginger, and lemongrass; cook and stir until brown, about 5 minutes.

3. Add crab legs and pepper. Cover and cook, tossing occasionally, for 15 minutes.

PER SERVING Calories: 208 | Fat: 8 g | Protein: 31 g | Sodium: 1,022 mg | Fiber: 0 g | Carbohydrate: 1 g

Mushroom Pork Medallions

You would never guess this meal is Paleo-approved. It tastes so amazing, you will swear it was deep fried with flour.

INGREDIENTS | SERVES 2

1 pound pork tenderloin
1 tablespoon olive oil
1 small onion, sliced
¼ cup sliced fresh mushrooms
1 garlic clove, minced
2 teaspoons flax meal
½ cup no-salt-added beef broth
¼ teaspoon dried rosemary, crushed
⅛ teaspoon ground black pepper

1. Slice tenderloin into ½" thick medallions.

2. In a skillet, heat olive oil over medium-high heat. Brown pork in oil for 2 minutes on each side.

3. Remove pork from skillet and set aside.

4. In same skillet, add onion, mushrooms, and garlic and sauté for 1 minute.

5. Stir in flax meal until blended.

6. Gradually stir in the broth, rosemary, and pepper. Bring to a boil; cook and stir for 1 minute or until thickened.

7. Lay pork medallions over mixture. Reduce heat; cover and simmer for 15 minutes or until meat juices run clear.

PER SERVING Calories: 196 | Fat: 11 g | Protein: 16 g | Sodium: 325 mg | Fiber: 1 g | Carbohydrate: 3.5 g

Citrus-Steamed Carrots

Figs are the fruit of gods and goddesses. Enjoy the pleasure yourself!

INGREDIENTS | SERVES 6

1 pound carrots

1 cup orange juice

2 tablespoons lemon juice

2 tablespoons lime juice

3 fresh figs

1 tablespoon extra-virgin olive oil

1 tablespoon capers

1. Peel and julienne the carrots. In a pot, combine the citrus juices and heat on medium-high. Add the carrots, cover, and steam until al dente. Remove from heat and let cool.

2. Cut the figs into wedges. Mound the carrots on serving plates and arrange the figs around the carrots. Sprinkle the olive oil and capers on top, and serve.

PER SERVING Calories: 93 | Fat: 2.5 g | Protein: 1.5 g | Sodium: 94 mg | Fiber: 3 g | Carbohydrate: 18 g

Mediterranean Green Beans

This simple recipe can be served hot or at room temperature.
Add any leftovers to salads as a nice healthy addition.

INGREDIENTS | SERVES 4

1 pound fresh green beans, ends trimmed, cut into 1" pieces

2 teaspoons minced fresh rosemary

1 teaspoon lemon zest

1 tablespoon olive oil

Freshly cracked black pepper, to taste

Taking Care of Your Produce

It is best to store unwashed fresh green beans in a plastic bag in the refrigerator. When you are ready to use the beans, wash them under cold running water. Washing fruits and vegetables right before you use them keeps them fresher and prevents mold from spoiling the final product.

1. Fill a medium-size saucepan with cold salted water and bring to a boil over high heat. Add the beans and cook until they are a vibrant green, just about 4 minutes.

2. Drain the beans and transfer to a large bowl. Add the remaining ingredients and toss to coat evenly. Serve warm or at room temperature.

PER SERVING Calories: 70 | Fat: 3.5 g | Protein: 2 g | Sodium: 22 mg | Fiber: 3.5 g | Carbohydrate: 9 g

Roasted Asparagus

Use thicker asparagus to withstand the heat of the grill.
Be sure to remove the woody end of the stalks first.

INGREDIENTS | **SERVES 6**

2 bunches asparagus
1 tablespoon extra-virgin olive oil
Lemon juice, to taste (optional)
Freshly cracked black pepper, to taste

Asparagus

Asparagus is low in calories and sodium, and offers numerous vitamins and minerals, most notably folate and potassium. The stalks also offer a blast of inflammation-fighting antioxidants.

Preheat grill to medium. Toss the asparagus in the oil, then drain on a rack and season with lemon juice and pepper. Grill the asparagus for 1 to 2 minutes on each side (cook to desired doneness). Serve immediately.

PER SERVING Calories: 30 | Fat: 2 g | Protein: 1 g | Sodium: 1 mg | Fiber: 1 g | Carbohydrate: 2 g

Roasted Peppers

Many people don't know that peppers become very sweet when roasted.

INGREDIENTS | SERVES 6

2 tablespoons olive oil
2 green peppers
2 yellow peppers
2 red peppers
6 cloves garlic, minced
Freshly cracked black pepper, to taste

1. Pour the olive oil in a stainless steel bowl. Dip the peppers in the olive oil, then roast or grill them on an open flame (reserve the bowl with the oil in it). Shock the peppers in ice water and remove the skins.

2. Julienne the peppers and add them to the bowl with the olive oil, along with the garlic and black pepper,.

3. Let sit at room temperature in serving bowl until ready to serve.

PER SERVING Calories: 76 | Fat: 4.5 g | Protein: 1.5 g | Sodium: 1 mg | Fiber: 2.5 g | Carbohydrate: 9 g

Roasted Kale

This is a simple recipe that yields a crisp, chewy kale that is irresistible. You can also slice up some collard greens or Swiss chard as a substitute for kale, or mix them all together for a tasty medley.

INGREDIENTS | SERVES 2

6 cups kale
1 tablespoon extra-virgin olive oil
1 teaspoon garlic powder

1. Preheat oven to 375°F.

2. Wash and trim kale by pulling leaves off the tough stems or running a sharp knife down the length of the stem.

3. Place leaves in a medium-size bowl; toss with extra-virgin olive oil and garlic powder.

4. Roast for 5 minutes; turn kale over and roast another 7–10 minutes, until kale turns brown and becomes paper-thin and brittle.

5. Remove from oven and serve immediately.

PER SERVING Calories: 160 | Fat: 8 g | Protein: 6 g | Sodium: 249 mg | Fiber: 4 g | Carbohydrate: 20 g

Dal

Dal is a classic East Indian dish. Now you can enjoy this excellent cuisine in the comfort of your own home!

INGREDIENTS | SERVES 6

6 cloves garlic

¼ Scotch bonnet chili pepper

1 tablespoon olive oil

1 cup dried yellow split peas

4 cups Basic Vegetable Stock (Chapter 11) or low-sodium canned vegetable stock

Caution: Hot

Scotch bonnet chili peppers are among the hottest peppers in the world. They are comparable to habanero peppers in terms of their hotness, but they have a flavor distinct from their habanero cousin's. If you want to cool this dish off a bit, use jalapeño peppers instead.

1. Mince the garlic. Stem, seed, and mince the chili pepper.

2. Heat the oil to medium temperature in a medium-size saucepot; sauté the garlic and chili for 1 minute.

3. Add the peas and stock; simmer for 1–2 hours, until the peas are thoroughly cooked. Serve with flatbread.

PER SERVING Calories: 143 | Fat: 1 g | Protein: 8 g | Sodium: 174 mg | Fiber: 8.5 g | Carbohydrate: 20 g

Spicy Chicken Burgers

You can substitute ground turkey or pork for the chicken. Adjust the quantity of pepper flakes to control the spiciness.

INGREDIENTS | SERVES 4

1 pound ground chicken breast
¼ cup finely chopped yellow onion
¼ cup finely chopped red bell pepper
1 teaspoon minced garlic
¼ cup thinly sliced scallions
½ teaspoon hot pepper flakes
Freshly cracked black pepper, to taste

1. Clean and oil broiler rack. Preheat broiler to medium.

2. Combine all the ingredients in a medium-size bowl, mixing lightly. Broil the burgers for 4–5 minutes per side until firm through the center and the juices run clear. Transfer to a plate and tent with tinfoil to keep warm. Allow to rest 1–2 minutes before serving.

PER SERVING Calories: 145 | Fat: 3 g | Protein: 27 g | Sodium: 20 mg | Fiber: 0 g | Carbohydrate: 1 g

Ginger-Orange Chicken Breast

This recipe is great chilled, sliced, and served on a crispy green salad.

INGREDIENTS | **SERVES 4**

4 (5-ounce) skinless, boneless chicken breasts
2 tablespoons olive oil
½ teaspoon seasoned salt
Freshly cracked black pepper, to taste
2 cloves garlic, minced
2 tablespoons grated ginger
2 teaspoons orange zest
½ cup 100 percent orange juice

Working with Chicken

Use fresh boneless, skinless breasts available in the meat section of your grocer. Use a good reputable brand and check the freshness date. Prior to cooking or preparing, always rinse the meat under cold running water and pat dry with paper towels.

1. Rinse the chicken under cold running water and pat dry with paper towels. Heat the olive oil in a small nonstick skillet over medium-high heat. Season the chicken with salt and pepper. Brown the chicken, turning it once, about 8 minutes per side. Transfer the chicken to a plate and keep warm.

2. Add the garlic to the pan and cook for about 1 minute, stirring frequently to prevent burning. Add the ginger, orange zest, and juice, and bring to a simmer. Add the chicken and any reserved juices and heat through, about 4–5 minutes. Cut through the bottom of the chicken to make sure it is cooked. Adjust seasoning to taste. Serve hot with the sauce.

PER SERVING Calories: 240 | Fat: 9.5 g | Protein: 34 g | Sodium: 138 mg | Fiber: 0 g | Carbohydrate: 3 g

CHAPTER 9

Snacks

Deviled Eggs

Eggs are a staple in the Paleolithic diet. This is a quick recipe that can be whipped up in no time. Kids and adults will love these and they can be easily served at parties or family gatherings.

INGREDIENTS | SERVES 10

10 large eggs, hard-boiled
2 green onions, finely chopped
2 cloves garlic, finely chopped
1 stalk celery, finely chopped
1 teaspoon mustard powder
1 teaspoon black pepper
Sweet paprika, to taste

1. Peel eggs, cut in half lengthwise, and separate yolks from whites.

2. Combine egg yolks, onions, garlic, celery, mustard powder, and black pepper. Mix well to form paste.

3. Stuff egg whites with yolk mixture.

4. Sprinkle paprika over eggs and serve.

PER SERVING Calories: 76 | Fat: 5 g | Protein: 7 g | Sodium: 63 mg | Fiber: 0 g | Carbohydrate: 1.5 g

Baked Apples

You will feel as if you're eating apple pie when you eat these and your house will smell like Thanksgiving dinner whenever you make them.

INGREDIENTS | SERVES 6

6 Pink Lady apples
1 cup unsweetened coconut flakes
Ground cinnamon, to taste

1. Preheat oven to 350°F.

2. Remove cores to ½" of the bottom of the apples.

3. Place apples in a medium baking dish.

4. Fill cores with coconut flakes and sprinkle with cinnamon.

5. Bake for 10–15 minutes. Apples are done when they are completely soft and brown on top.

PER SERVING Calories: 159 | Fat: 9.5 g | Protein: 1 g | Sodium: 6.5 mg | Fiber: 4.5 g | Carbohydrate: 21 g

Sardines in Red Pepper Cups

These cups can be put together in a few minutes and are ideal snacks for transporting. Additionally, this recipe is a great source of omega-3.

INGREDIENTS | **SERVES 1**

1 (3.75-ounce) can no-salt-added, skinless, boneless sardines

1 red pepper

Juice of 1 lemon

Black pepper, to taste

1. Open and drain container of sardines.

2. Cut red pepper in half, remove ribs and seeds, and fill with sardines.

3. Sprinkle with lemon juice and pepper.

PER SERVING Calories: 187 | Fat: 8.5 g | Protein: 19 g | Sodium: 377 mg | Fiber: 2 g | Carbohydrate: 8 g

Whey Protein Smoothie

This protein smoothie is the perfect post-workout meal. You will feel refreshed and satisfied after drinking this replenishment meal. Feel free to experiment with fruit of your choice.

INGREDIENTS | SERVES 1

1 scoop whey protein, any flavor

1 tablespoon nut butter of your choice (almond, macadamia, or sunflower)

2 tablespoons cacao nibs

8 ounces coconut water

1 frozen sliced banana (or fruit of your choice)

Combine all ingredients into blender. Blend and enjoy.

PER SERVING Calories: 434 | Fat: 18 g | Protein: 7.5 g | Sodium: 291 mg | Fiber: 6.5 g | Carbohydrate: 67 g

Smoothies and Shakes

Smoothies are a staple for athletes. They are great for after a workout, because they can be mixed quickly in water. If you are replacing lost electrolytes, you should consider drinking coconut water post workout or race. Coconuts are an all-natural supply of electrolytes, unlike commercially sold high-sugar electrolyte drinks that can leave you more thirsty after consumption.

Broccoli, Pine Nut, and Apple Salad

This quick little salad will tide you over to your next meal. The broccoli and apple taste great together and the toasted pine nuts add a little bit of crunch.

INGREDIENTS | SERVES 2

4 tablespoons olive oil
¾ cup pine nuts
2 cups broccoli florets
2 cups diced green apples
Juice of 1 lemon

1. Heat olive oil in a small frying pan and sauté the pine nuts until golden brown.

2. Mix broccoli and apples in a medium bowl. Add the pine nuts and toss.

3. Squeeze lemon juice over salad and serve.

PER SERVING Calories: 621 | Fat: 53 g | Protein: 15 g | Sodium: 34 mg | Fiber: 7 g | Carbohydrate: 31 g

Cinnamon Toasted Butternut Squash

This side dish or snack is a great fall dish. It smells amazing and will give you the carbohydrate boost your glycogen storage needs.

INGREDIENTS | **SERVES 4**

3 cups butternut squash, cubed

1 tablespoon ground cinnamon

1 teaspoon nutmeg

1. Preheat oven to 350°F.

2. Place squash in 9" × 11" baking dish. Sprinkle with cinnamon and nutmeg.

3. Bake for 30 minutes or until tender and slightly brown.

PER SERVING Calories: 48 | Fat: 0 g | Protein: 1 g | Sodium: 4 mg | Fiber: 2 g | Carbohydrate: 13 g

Red Pepper and Fennel Salad

Fennel has a fantastic licorice flavor that blends nicely with nuts. The red pepper adds a flash of color and a bit of sweetness to the mix.

INGREDIENTS | SERVES 1

⅓ cup pine nuts, toasted

3 tablespoons sesame seeds, toasted

2 tablespoons olive oil

1 medium red bell pepper, halved; seeds and ribs removed

6 leaves romaine lettuce, shredded

½ bulb fennel, diced

1 tablespoon walnut oil

Juice from 1 lime

Black pepper, to taste

Walnut Oil

Walnut oil cannot withstand high heat, so it's best to add it to food that has been cooked or is served raw, such as a salad. If you choose to cook with it, use a lower flame to avoid burning the oil.

1. Preheat broiler.

2. In a medium skillet, sauté pine nuts and sesame seeds in olive oil over medium heat for 5 minutes.

3. Grill pepper under the broiler until the skin is blackened, and the flesh has softened slightly.

4. Place pepper halves in a paper bag to cool slightly. When cool enough to handle, remove skin and slice into strips.

5. Combine red pepper slices, lettuce, and fennel in a salad bowl.

6. Add walnut oil, lime juice, and black pepper to taste. Mix well with salad bowl contents. Add nut mixture and serve.

PER SERVING Calories: 1,221 | Fat: 121 g | Protein: 19 g | Sodium: 81 mg | Fiber: 11 g | Carbohydrate: 27 g

Shrimp Cocktail

Shrimp is another flavorful, low-fat shellfish that is a nice addition to the Paleolithic lifestyle.

INGREDIENTS | **SERVES 4**

6 tablespoons horseradish root, grated

1 tablespoon raw honey

1 (6-ounce) can organic no-salt-added tomato paste

Juice of 1 lemon

½ teaspoon red pepper flakes

1 pound jumbo cooked shrimp, peeled

In a small bowl, blend the horseradish, honey, tomato paste, lemon juice, and red pepper flakes. Serve immediately with jumbo shrimp.

PER SERVING Calories: 152 | Fat: 2 g | Protein: 19 g | Sodium: 238 mg | Fiber: 3 g | Carbohydrate: 16 g

Shrimp Facts

Shrimp is a great protein source. A single (4-ounce) serving of shrimp contains 24 grams of protein with less than 1 gram of fat. It contains a high level of selenium, vitamin D, and vitamin B_{12}. Selenium has been linked with cancer-fighting properties and is utilized in DNA repair.

Floret Salad

Broccoli is one of the most nutrient dense green vegetables. Try this floret salad to maximize on taste while boosting your health simultaneously.

INGREDIENTS | SERVES 2

⅔ cup fresh cauliflower florets

⅔ cup fresh broccoli florets

2 tablespoons chopped red onion

8 ounces uncured nitrate-free bacon, cooked and chopped

5 teaspoons raw honey

¼ cup walnut oil

2 tablespoons whole cashews

1. In a medium bowl, combine cauliflower, broccoli, red onion, and bacon.

2. In a small bowl, whisk raw honey and walnut oil.

3. Combine honey mixture with florets and toss.

4. Top with cashews just before serving.

PER SERVING Calories: 930 | Fat: 79 g | Protein: 35 g | Sodium: 1,299 mg | Fiber: 2 g | Carbohydrate: 22 g

Broccoli: Superfood

Broccoli is one of the healthiest vegetables you can eat. Ounce for ounce, broccoli has more vitamin C than an orange and as much calcium as a glass of milk. Broccoli is packed with fiber to promote digestive health and it is quite rich in vitamin A.

Crunchy Fruit Salad

When you're in the mood for a sweet treat, this crunchy salad will fulfill that sugar craving and replenish glycogen storage post workouts.

INGREDIENTS | SERVES 2

½ fresh pineapple, peeled, cored, and cubed

1 medium fresh papaya, cubed

1 medium ripe banana, sliced

½ cup halved seedless grapes

1 tablespoon raw honey

¼ cup chopped cashews

¼ cup unsweetened coconut flakes

Combine all ingredients, toss, and serve.

PER SERVING Calories: 346 | Fat: 16 g | Protein: 6 g | Sodium: 11 mg | Fiber: 6.5 g | Carbohydrate: 53 g

Seasonal Fruits

It is always best to eat foods that are native to your area and in season. If you eat fruits that are imported they have traveled long distances and their freshness factor cannot be guaranteed. Your hunter-gather ancestors only had foods that were in season at the time of the hunt. They did not have the luxury of importing fruits from a neighboring area. Your body is made to change with the seasons.

Blueberry Antioxidant Smoothie

Blueberries contain one of the highest antioxidant levels found in fruit. This smoothie is refreshing while fighting free-radical oxidation in your body.

INGREDIENTS | SERVES 1

1 cup frozen blueberries
½ avocado
1 cup vanilla-flavored almond milk
⅛ teaspoon ground nutmeg
4–6 ice cubes

Combine all ingredients in a blender and purée until smooth.

PER SERVING Calories: 329 | Fat: 17 g | Protein: 13 g | Sodium: 141 mg | Fiber: 11 g | Carbohydrate: 39 g

Almond Joy Smoothie

This chocolate and coconut smoothie is a real treat when you are craving something sweet.

INGREDIENTS | **SERVES 1**

1 cup coconut milk

½ cup cacao nibs

3 tablespoons raw honey

½ teaspoon cinnamon

¼ teaspoon nutmeg

4–6 ice cubes

Combine all ingredients in a blender and purée until smooth.

PER SERVING Calories: 790 | Fat: 56 g | Protein: 5 g | Sodium: 32 mg | Fiber: 0 g | Carbohydrate: 79 g

Edamame

Edamame are fresh soybeans. You can eat them as a snack before sushi or as part of a crudités platter. Edamame are also an excellent addition to salads, soups, and rice dishes.

INGREDIENTS | **SERVES 6**

6 cups of water
½ teaspoon lemon juice
1 pound frozen edamame in pods

Snacks Should Be Healthful and Fun

Tastes are formed early. If your kids don't try something, don't make an issue, but keep presenting the food and see what happens. If you have a few kids in the house, have a "crunch contest"! Whose bite of celery or carrot or cucumber makes the loudest crunch? Everybody wins!

1. Bring the water and the lemon juice to a boil in a saucepan.

2. Add the edamame and let the water come back to a boil.

3. Cook on medium-high for 5 minutes.

4. Drain the edamame and rinse with cold water.

5. Drain again and serve either warm or cool.

PER SERVING Calories: 107 | Fat: 5 g | Protein: 9 g | Sodium: 204 mg | Fiber: 3 g | Carbohydrate: 8.5 g

Fresh Pepper Salsa

Tomatoes are a great source of the antioxidant vitamin C. You can also get creative and make your salsa with other vegetables, fruits, and spices.

INGREDIENTS | YIELDS 1 PINT

1 yellow bell pepper
1 orange bell pepper
1 or 2 poblano chilies
2 Anaheim chilies
1 or 2 jalapeño peppers
2 cloves garlic
¼ of a red onion
Juice of ½ lime
Freshly crushed black pepper, to taste
Canola oil (enough to coat the pan)
Cilantro, chopped, to taste (optional)

1. Place all ingredients (except the oil) in a food processor and pulse until desired chunkiness results. Taste and adjust for saltiness and heat.

2. In a medium pot, heat oil until slightly smoking. Add blended pepper mixture. Cook on high for 8–10 minutes, stirring occasionally. Sprinkle some chopped cilantro on top, if desired. Serve hot, cold, or at room temperature with tortilla chips, as a garnish for fish or poultry, or in your favorite burrito.

PER SERVING Calories: 104 | Fat: 1 g | Protein: 3 g | Sodium: 6 mg | Fiber: 6 g | Carbohydrate: 23 g

CHAPTER 10

Children's Favorites

Chicken Nuggets

These chicken nuggets are fantastic for kids and adults. Mix them in a green salad or serve with sweet potato fries.

INGREDIENTS | SERVES 4

2 boneless skinless chicken breasts, cut into bite-size pieces
½ cup olive oil
4 cloves garlic, minced
¼ teaspoon pepper
½ cup almond flour

1. Place chicken in shallow dish.

2. In small bowl, mix olive oil, garlic, and pepper.

3. Pour over chicken and marinate for 30 minutes in the refrigerator.

4. Preheat oven to 475°F.

5. Place almond flour in a shallow bowl.

6. Remove chicken from marinade and dredge in almond flour to coat.

7. Bake for 10 minutes or until brown.

PER SERVING Calories: 369 | Fat: 28 g | Protein: 20 g | Sodium: 2 mg | Fiber: 2 g | Carbohydrate: 12 g

Blueberry Cookie Balls

These antioxidant-packed cookie balls are a great alternative to commercial cookies. They taste great, are all natural, and will give your kids energy from all macronutrient categories.

INGREDIENTS | SERVES 12

2 egg whites

5 cups blueberries

4 teaspoons cinnamon

1½ teaspoons ginger

¼ cup raw honey

1 teaspoon vanilla extract

Glycemic Load and Kids

It is particularly important to limit children's sugar intake, because they are more sensitive to mood changes than adults and lack the ability to control their emotions. Recipes that contain fat, protein, and carbohydrates together minimize blood sugar spikes and pitfalls.

1. Whisk egg whites in a bowl until frothy.

2. Add all other ingredients and mix well.

3. Scoop out tablespoons of dough and form into balls. Place balls on a cookie sheet.

4. Cook in 350°F oven for 12–15 minutes.

5. Place on pan and chill in refrigerator for 1 hour.

PER SERVING Calories: 60 | Fat: 0.5 g | Protein: 1.5 g | Sodium: 12 mg | Fiber: 1.5 g | Carbohydrate: 14 g

Old-Fashioned Sweet Potato Hash Browns

These sweet potato hash browns are likely to become a family favorite. They are easy to make and packed with flavor your entire family will love.

INGREDIENTS | SERVES 6

3 tablespoons coconut oil

3 medium sweet potatoes, peeled and grated

1 tablespoon cinnamon

1. Heat the coconut oil in large sauté pan over medium-high heat.

2. Cook sweet potatoes in hot oil for 7 minutes, stirring often.

3. Once brown, sprinkle with cinnamon and serve.

PER SERVING Calories: 116 | Fat: 7 g | Protein: 1.5 g | Sodium: 36 mg | Fiber: 2 g | Carbohydrate: 13 g

Turkey Lettuce Wrap

Turkey is a low-fat protein source that kids are sure to love. Although these wraps are a bit more complex to make, you can make a larger batch of the filling and serve it over salad at a later meal.

INGREDIENTS | SERVES 4

3 tablespoons walnut oil
3 shallots, chopped
1 piece lemongrass, thinly sliced
1 serrano chili pepper, thinly sliced
½ teaspoon fresh ground black pepper
1½ pounds ground turkey
⅓ cup fresh lime juice
2 tablespoons sesame oil
4 tablespoons coconut oil
½ cup Thai basil leaves, thinly sliced
8 large butter lettuce leaves

1. In a large skillet, heat walnut oil over medium heat.

2. Add shallots, lemongrass, serrano pepper, and black pepper. Cook until the shallots soften, about 4 minutes.

3. Add ground turkey and stir frequently until cooked through, approximately 8–10 minutes.

4. Add lime juice, sesame oil, and coconut oil and cook for 1 minute.

5. Turn the heat off and mix in basil leaves.

6. Wrap mixture in lettuce leaves and serve.

PER SERVING Calories: 381 | Fat: 29 g | Protein: 40 g | Sodium: 1 mg | Fiber: 1 g | Carbohydrate: 1 g

Paleo Stuffed Peppers

Peppers are chockfull of great vitamins and minerals that kids need. These peppers are so fun to eat, they won't know how healthy they are.

INGREDIENTS | SERVES 4

4 red bell peppers

2 tablespoons olive oil

3 cloves garlic, chopped

1 onion, chopped

1 pound ground chicken

2 green bell peppers, chopped

1 cup celery, diced

1 cup mushrooms, sliced

2 tablespoons chili powder

1 tablespoon cumin

1 (28-ounce) can organic, no-salt-added diced tomatoes

1 (6-ounce) can organic, no-salt-added tomato paste

1. Cut off tops of red peppers and remove seeds and ribs. Set aside.

2. In skillet, heat olive oil, and sauté garlic and onion for 2 minutes.

3. Add ground chicken and cook until browned, about 5 minutes.

4. Add green peppers, celery, mushrooms, chili powder, and cumin and continue cooking for 5 minutes.

5. Stuff mixture into red peppers and place in slow cooker.

6. Pour diced tomatoes and tomato paste over peppers and cook on high for 5 hours.

PER SERVING Calories: 298 | Fat: 13 g | Protein: 22 g | Sodium: 553 mg | Fiber: 7 g | Carbohydrate: 29 g

Paleo Chocolate Bars

Your kids will be thrilled when they see these chocolate bars in their lunch boxes. These bars are quick to whip up and quick to eat. The amount of honey can be varied depending on your desired sweetness level.

INGREDIENTS | SERVES 8

1 tablespoon raw honey
4 tablespoons coconut oil
¼ cup ground almonds
¼ cup ground hazelnuts
¼ cup sunflower seeds
¼ cup cacao powder
¾ cups shredded unsweetened coconut flakes

Natural Sugars

Although natural honey is an acceptable Paleolithic diet food, you should still eat it in moderation. It does cause an increase in blood sugar levels, thus a spike in insulin.

1. Melt honey and coconut oil in saucepan over medium heat.

2. In a mixing bowl, combine almonds, hazelnuts, sunflower seeds, cacao powder, and coconut. Mix thoroughly.

3. Add honey mixture to bowl and mix well.

4. Pour dough into an 8" × 8" baking pan and store in refrigerator or freezer until firm, about 10 minutes.

5. Cut into squares and enjoy.

PER SERVING Calories: 154 | Fat: 15 g | Protein: 2 g | Sodium: 2 mg | Fiber: 2 g | Carbohydrate: 5 g

Kids' Favorite Trail Mix

For kids who love potato chips, this recipe will be a nice alternative.
It has a sweet and salty taste to satisfy all their cravings.

INGREDIENTS | SERVES 8

½ cup cashews
½ cup almonds
½ cup macadamia nuts
½ cup pistachio nuts
4 tablespoons raw honey
1 teaspoon sea salt
½ teaspoon ground black pepper
¼ teaspoon ground cumin
1 teaspoon curry powder
1 pinch ground cloves
1 teaspoon ground cinnamon

1. Preheat oven to 300°F.

2. Place all nuts on a large baking sheet and bake for 10–12 minutes, taking care they do not burn. Remove from oven and let cool approximately 5 minutes.

3. In a small bowl, mix honey, salt, pepper, cumin, curry powder, cloves, and cinnamon.

4. In a large saucepan over medium heat, place the nuts and half of the honey mixture. When the mixture begins to melt, mix in the remaining honey mixture.

5. Shake the pan until all the nuts are coated, about 5 minutes.

6. Cool on wax paper. Use a spoon to separate nuts that stick together.

PER SERVING Calories: 207 | Fat: 16 g | Protein: 5 g | Sodium: 292 mg | Fiber: 2.5 g | Carbohydrate: 15 g

Tuna Salad

Tuna is a common family favorite. This Paleolithic diet salad recipe is sure to be a pleaser, too. With the addition of fresh mint and parsley, your taste buds will surely smile.

INGREDIENTS | SERVES 2

1 (6-ounce) can no-salt-added tuna in water, drained

20 cherry tomatoes, halved

1 cucumber, peeled and chopped

4 green onions, chopped

¼ cup olive oil

¼ cup lemon juice

4 cloves garlic, minced

¼ cup chopped fresh parsley

¼ cup chopped fresh mint leaves

In a large serving bowl, combine all ingredients and mix well. Serve chilled.

PER SERVING Calories: 385 | Fat: 28 g | Protein: 25 g | Sodium: 296 mg | Fiber: 2.5 g | Carbohydrate: 11 g

Mercury and Children

Children under the age of six should not eat tuna, swordfish, shark, king mackerel, or marlin due to high levels of mercury in their flesh. As an alternative, young children should eat fish lower on the food chain such as tilapia, cod, halibut, and snapper.

Roasted Spicy Pumpkin Seeds

This spicy seed recipe is sure to be a favorite with the family for snacking. They are quick to prepare and easy to grab for on the go snacks.

INGREDIENTS | SERVES 6

3 cups raw pumpkin seeds
½ cup olive oil
½ teaspoon garlic powder
Ground black pepper, to taste

Pumpkin Seed Benefits

Pumpkin seeds have great health benefits. They contain L-tryptophan, a compound found to naturally fight depression and they are high in zinc, a mineral that protects against osteoporosis.

1. Preheat oven to 300°F.

2. In a medium bowl, mix together the pumpkin seeds, olive oil, garlic powder, and black pepper until the pumpkin seeds are evenly coated.

3. Spread in an even layer on a cookie sheet.

4. Bake for 1 hour and 15 minutes, stirring every 10–15 minutes until toasted.

PER SERVING Calories: 532 | Fat: 50 g | Protein: 17 g | Sodium: 13 mg | Fiber: 3 g | Carbohydrate: 12 g

Apricot Banana Smoothie

Apricot and banana together make a delicious and refreshing smoothie.

INGREDIENTS	SERVES 1

3 fresh apricots, pitted and diced

1 banana, diced

1 cup coconut milk

4 teaspoons raw honey

4–6 ice cubes

Combine all ingredients in blender and blend until smooth and frosty.

PER SERVING Calories: 544 | Fat: 30 g | Protein: 5 g | Sodium: 22 mg | Fiber: 9 g | Carbohydrate: 76 g

Apricots Are Quite Beneficial

Apricots are often overlooked as a fruit choice, but these little tangy fruits are an excellent source of vitamins A, C, and E, potassium, and iron. You could fulfill almost 50 percent of your vitamin A daily value with three apricots a day.

Grass-Fed Lamb Meatballs

Meatballs are always a kid favorite. These grass-fed lamb meatballs are high in good fats that contribute to their taste and their health factor.

INGREDIENTS | SERVES 6

¼ cup pine nuts

4 tablespoons olive oil, divided

1½ pounds ground grass-fed lamb

¼ cup minced garlic

2 tablespoons cumin

1. Over medium-high heat sauté pine nuts in 2 tablespoons olive oil for 2 minutes until brown. Remove from pan and allow to cool.

2. In a large bowl, combine lamb, garlic, cumin, and pine nuts and form into meatballs.

3. Add remaining olive oil to pan and fry meatballs until cooked through, about 5–10 minutes, depending on size of meatballs.

PER SERVING Calories: 148 | Fat: 13 g | Protein: 5 g | Sodium: 201 mg | Fiber: 2.5 g | Carbohydrate: 6.5 g

CHAPTER 11

Soups and Starters

Basic Chicken Soup

The major advantage of this soup is that it will be much lower in sodium than other canned chicken soups. The only limit is your imagination. Each time you make it, substitute different vegetables and seasonings to tantalize your taste buds.

INGREDIENTS | SERVES 6

5–6 pounds chicken (including giblets)
2 medium carrots
2 stalks celery
4 large yellow onions
¼ bunch parsley
12 cups water
Freshly cracked black pepper, to taste
Kosher salt, to taste

Don't Cry over Cut Onions

The sulfur in onions can cause the tears to flow. To avoid teary eyes, peel onions under cold water to wash away the volatile sulfur compounds. Onions are worth it, since they have anti-inflammatory effects on the joints.

1. Clean, trim, and quarter the chicken. Peel and chop all the vegetables. Chop parsley.

2. Place the chicken and giblets in a stockpot, add the water, and bring to a boil. Reduce heat to a simmer and skim off all foam.

3. Add all the remaining ingredients and simmer uncovered for about 3 hours.

4. Remove the chicken and giblets from the stockpot; discard giblets. Remove the meat from the bones, discard the bones, and return the meat to the broth; serve.

PER SERVING Calories: 183 | Fat: 8 g | Protein: 16 g | Sodium: 84 mg | Fiber: 1.5 g | Carbohydrate: 5.5 g

Basic Vegetable Stock

Another great broth that is low on sodium and high on disease-fighting phytochemicals. Try adding mushrooms for additional flavor.

INGREDIENTS | YIELDS 1 GALLON; SERVING SIZE 1 CUP

2 pounds yellow onions
1 pound carrots
1 pound celery
1 bunch fresh parley stems
1½ gallons water
4 stems fresh thyme
2 bay leaves (fresh or dried)
10–20 peppercorns

Homemade Stocks

Your homemade stocks give a special quality to all the dishes you add them to. Not only will the flavor of homemade stocks be better than that from purchased bases, but you will have added your own personal touch to the meal. Always cook them uncovered, as covering will cause them to become cloudy.

1. Peel and roughly chop the onions and carrots. Roughly chop the celery (stalks only; no leaves) and fresh parsley stems.

2. Put the vegetables and water in a stockpot over medium heat; bring to a simmer and cook, uncovered, for 1½ hours.

3. Add the herbs and peppercorns, and continue to simmer, uncovered, for 45 minutes. Adjust seasonings to taste as necessary.

4. Remove from heat and cool by submerging the pot in a bath of ice and water. Place in freezer-safe containers and store in the freezer until ready to use.

PER SERVING Calories: 22 | Fat: 0 g | Protein: 0 g | Sodium: 31 mg | Fiber: 0 g | Carbohydrate: 5.3 g

Butternut Squash Soup

*This soup is a scrumptious treat on a cool fall day. Warm family
and friends with a delightful blend of aroma and flavor.*

INGREDIENTS | SERVES 4

1 tablespoon olive oil

1 medium onion, chopped

1 pound butternut squash, peeled,
seeded, and chopped

½ cup flax meal

32 ounces organic low-sodium chicken
broth

1 cup almond milk

½ teaspoon ground cinnamon

¼ teaspoon ground cloves

¼ teaspoon ground nutmeg

1. In a soup pot or Dutch oven, heat olive oil over
   medium-high heat. Sauté onion and butternut squash
   in oil for 5 minutes.

2. Add flax meal and chicken broth, and increase heat
   to high.

3. Bring to a boil, then turn to low, and simmer for 45
   minutes.

4. In batches, purée squash mixture in blender or food
   processor and return to pot.

5. Stir in almond milk, cinnamon, cloves, and nutmeg.

PER SERVING Calories: 182 | Fat: 9 g | Protein: 8.5 g |
Sodium: 495 mg | Fiber: 5.5 g | Carbohydrate: 20 g

Cream of Cauliflower Soup

Cauliflower is a fantastic vegetable in Paleolithic diet recipes. Blended cauliflower can be used as a thickener in recipes that normally called for potatoes or root vegetables. Best of all, cauliflower won't spike your insulin levels.

INGREDIENTS | **SERVES 4**

1 large head cauliflower, chopped
3 stalks celery, chopped
1 carrot, chopped
2 cloves garlic, minced
1 onion, chopped
2 teaspoons ground cumin
½ teaspoon ground black pepper
1 tablespoon chopped parsley
¼ teaspoon dill

1. In a soup pot or Dutch oven, combine cauliflower, celery, carrot, garlic, onions, cumin, and pepper.

2. Add water to just cover ingredients in pot. Bring to a boil over high heat.

3. Reduce heat to low. Simmer about 8 minutes or until vegetables are tender.

4. Stir in parsley and dill before serving.

PER SERVING Calories: 56 | Fat: 0.5 g | Protein: 3 g | Sodium: 83 mg | Fiber: 5 g | Carbohydrate: 10 g

Gazpacho

Gazpacho is best made the day before so that the flavors will penetrate all the vegetables. It should be served chilled.

INGREDIENTS | SERVES 6

1 (28-ounce) can chopped tomatoes, no salt added

1 green bell pepper, chopped

3 medium tomatoes, peeled and chopped

1 cucumber, peeled and chopped

1 small onion, chopped

2 tablespoons olive oil

½ teaspoon black pepper

½ teaspoon paprika

¼ teaspoon cayenne pepper

1 teaspoon chopped chives

2 teaspoons chopped parsley

½ clove garlic, minced

4½ teaspoons lemon juice

1. Blend canned tomatoes in blender until smooth. Pour into large bowl.

2. Add remaining ingredients to bowl.

3. Refrigerate at least 12 hours, then serve.

PER SERVING Calories: 113 | Fat: 5 g | Protein: 3 g | Sodium: 297 mg | Fiber: 3.5 g | Carbohydrate: 15 g

Scallion Chive Soup

Chive is a member of the onion family. It adds a sweet, mild oniony taste to recipes.

INGREDIENTS | SERVES 2

3 teaspoons olive oil
½ cup shredded zucchini
½ cup chopped shallots
1 clove garlic, minced
1 cup chopped scallions
½ cup chopped chives
2 cups no-salt-added chicken broth
½ cup water

Chive as Insect Repellant

Chive has such a strong scent that it can be used in gardens as an insect repellant. Garlic has also been known to be an effective defense against pests.

1. Heat olive oil in a soup pot or Dutch oven over medium-low heat. Cook zucchini, shallots, and garlic in oil for 3–5 minutes.

2. Add scallions and chives and cook for 2 minutes more.

3. Add chicken broth and water. Increase heat to high and bring to a boil.

4. Reduce heat to low and simmer for 5 minutes.

5. In batches, purée soup in blender or food processor.

PER SERVING Calories: 130 | Fat: 7 g | Protein: 6 g | Sodium: 568 mg | Fiber: 2.5 g | Carbohydrate: 12 g

Scallop Ceviche

This recipe calls for overnight preparation, so plan accordingly.

INGREDIENTS | SERVES 8

2 pounds small bay scallops

1 cup lime juice

1 large onion, chopped

20 black olives

½ cup water

3 medium tomatoes, peeled and diced

½ cup olive oil

1 teaspoon oregano

⅛ teaspoon white or black pepper

1. Marinate scallops in lime juice for 3 to 4 hours.

2. Drain and rinse scallops in cold water.

3. Place scallops in a medium bowl and add remaining ingredients. Mix and store overnight in refrigerator.

4. Serve chilled.

PER SERVING Calories: 163 | Fat: 3.5 g | Protein: 27 g | Sodium: 494 mg | Fiber: 1.5 g | Carbohydrate: 4.5 g

Eating Raw Food

Many people advocate eating only raw food. However, you should be aware that many illnesses and parasites caused by bacteria and small organisms are killed by cooking food. Eating uncooked food is a risk, no matter how tasty the dish.

Chopped Chicken Livers

Organ meat is a great source of protein, vitamin A, and the mineral iron. If chicken liver is not to your liking, you might want to try beef liver, which has more vitamins and minerals and less fat calories per gram.

INGREDIENTS | SERVES 4

1 pound chicken livers, trimmed
2 medium onions, chopped
¼ cup olive oil
½ teaspoon ground black pepper
2 hard-boiled eggs, peeled and chopped

1. Preheat broiler. Place chicken livers on a cookie sheet.

2. Broil chicken livers, turning frequently, for 8–10 minutes, or until cooked thoroughly and no longer pink inside.

3. In large skillet, heat olive oil over medium heat. Sauté onions 10 minutes, or until browned.

4. Place chicken livers, onions, and pepper in food processor and pulse until coarsely chopped. Pour mixture into a medium bowl.

5. Fold eggs into liver mixture.

PER SERVING Calories: 274 | Fat: 18 g | Protein: 36 g | Sodium: 121 mg | Fiber: 0 g | Carbohydrate: 6 g

Scallops Wrapped in Bacon

This common party appetizer has been revamped for Paleo with nitrate-free bacon.
You are sure to like these much better than the old unhealthy version.

INGREDIENTS | SERVES 10

2 tablespoons olive oil
20 large scallops
2 tablespoons garlic, minced
20 slices uncured, nitrate-free bacon

1. Heat olive oil in a large frying pan over medium-high heat. Sauté scallops in oil with garlic until scallops are lightly browned. Set aside to cool.

2. Cook bacon slightly on each side and use to wrap scallops. Make sure bacon is not overcooked or it will not wrap around scallops.

3. Secure each appetizer with a toothpick and serve warm.

PER SERVING Calories: 159 | Fat: 15 g | Protein: 13 g | Sodium: 291 mg | Fiber: 0 g | Carbohydrate: 0 g

Sautéed Brussels Sprouts

Brussels sprouts will no longer be boring when they are spiced up with bacon and garlic. These are a great appetizer or side dish for any main meal.

INGREDIENTS | SERVES 4

4 cups fresh Brussels sprouts

2 tablespoons olive oil

½ cup minced shallots

½ cup sliced mushrooms

4 cloves garlic, minced

3 ounces uncured, nitrate-free bacon, diced

1. Steam Brussels sprouts until tender, about 10 minutes.

2. Heat olive oil in a medium frying pan over medium heat. Sauté shallots, mushrooms, and garlic until caramelized, approximately 5 minutes. Remove from pan.

3. In the same pan, cook bacon until crisp.

4. Add Brussels sprouts and shallot mixture to bacon and cook over medium heat for 5 minutes. Remove from heat and serve.

PER SERVING Calories: 141 | Fat: 7.5 g | Protein: 5 g | Sodium: 37 mg | Fiber: 4 g | Carbohydrate: 19 g

Stuffed Mushroom Caps

These appetizers are a bit more exciting than traditional bread crumb recipes. They are stuffed with protein and fats to ensure more macronutrients in each bite.

INGREDIENTS | SERVES 10

20 button mushrooms
2 tablespoons walnut oil
½ cup finely chopped walnuts
½ pound chopped ground turkey
4 cloves garlic, minced
½ teaspoon black pepper

1. Preheat oven to 350°F.

2. Remove stems and hollow out mushroom caps. Dice mushroom stems and place in medium bowl.

3. Heat walnut oil in a medium frying pan and cook ground turkey and garlic for 5–8 minutes, or until turkey is no longer pink.

4. Add mushrooms, nuts, and pepper to the ground turkey and cook until mushrooms are soft, about 8 minutes.

5. Stuff turkey mixture into mushroom caps and place on cookie sheet.

6. Bake 20 minutes or until golden brown on top.

PER SERVING Calories: 88 | Fat: 7 g | Protein: 7 g | Sodium: 2 mg | Fiber: 1 g | Carbohydrate: 2 g

Tomato Soup

Tomato soup is one of the most famous comfort foods. This recipe is not made with cream or butter, yet has an old fashioned taste you'll love.

INGREDIENTS | SERVES 4

4 cups chopped fresh tomatoes

1 slice onion

4 whole cloves

2 cups organic, no-salt-added chicken broth

2 tablespoons olive oil

2 tablespoons almond flour

Juice from 1 lime

1. In a stockpot, over medium heat, combine the tomatoes, onion, cloves, and chicken broth.

2. Bring to a boil, and gently boil for about 20 minutes to blend all of the flavors.

3. Remove from heat and strain into large bowl. Discard solids.

4. In the now-empty stockpot, combine olive oil with almond flour. Stir until the mixture thickens.

5. Gradually whisk in tomato mixture to avoid clumps. Add lime to taste.

PER SERVING Calories: 113 | Fat: 7 g | Protein: 4 g | Sodium: 286 mg | Fiber: 2 g | Carbohydrate: 10 g

Carrot-Lemon Soup

This is a great anytime soup and can be served either hot or cold.

INGREDIENTS | SERVES 6

2 pounds carrots

2 large yellow onions

2 cloves garlic

1 fresh lemon

3 tablespoons olive oil

1 teaspoon fresh minced ginger

6 cups Basic Vegetable Stock (see this chapter) or low-sodium canned vegetable stock

Freshly cracked black pepper, to taste

3 fresh scallions, for garnish

1. Peel and dice the carrots and onions. Mince the garlic. Juice and grate the lemon.

2. Heat the oil to medium in a large stockpot and lightly sauté the carrots, onions, and garlic.

3. Add the stock and simmer for approximately 1 hour. Add the ginger, lemon juice, and zest. Season with pepper.

4. Chill and serve with finely chopped scallions as garnish.

PER SERVING Calories: 153 | Fat: 7 g | Protein: 3 g | Sodium: 62 mg | Fiber: 5 g | Carbohydrate: 16 g

Lemon Know-How

The thought of lemons may make your cheeks pucker, but it's well worth the powerful dose of cold-fighting vitamin C. The average lemon contains approximately 3 tablespoons of juice. Allow lemons to come to room temperature before squeezing to maximize the amount of juice extracted.

Pumpkin Soup

This is a perfect autumn soup to celebrate the harvest season. If you're short on time or pumpkins are out of season, substitute 1 (15-ounce) can of puréed pumpkin for the fresh pumpkin.

INGREDIENTS | **SERVES 6**

2 cups large-diced fresh sugar pumpkin, seeds reserved separately

3 leeks, sliced

1½ teaspoons minced fresh ginger

1 tablespoon olive oil

½ teaspoon grated fresh lemon zest

1 teaspoon fresh lemon juice

2 quarts Basic Vegetable Stock (see this chapter) or low-sodium canned vegetable stock

Freshly ground black pepper, to taste

1 tablespoon extra-virgin olive oil, for drizzling

Zesting

If you don't have a zester, you can still easily make lemon zest. Simply use your cheese grater, but be careful to grate only the rind and not the white pith, which tends to be bitter.

1. Preheat oven to 375°F.

2. Clean the pumpkin seeds thoroughly, place them on a baking sheet, and sprinkle with salt. Roast for approximately 5–8 minutes, until light golden.

3. Place the diced pumpkin in a baking dish with the leeks, ginger, and olive oil; roast for 45 minutes to 1 hour, until cooked al dente.

4. Transfer the cooked pumpkin mixture to a large stockpot and add the zest, juice, stock, and pepper; let simmer for 30–45 minutes.

5. To serve, ladle into serving bowls. Drizzle with extra-virgin olive oil and sprinkle with toasted pumpkin seeds.

PER SERVING Calories: 100 | Fat: 4 g | Protein: 3 g | Sodium: 62 mg | Fiber: 1.5 g | Carbohydrate: 10 g

Entertaining and Parties

Paleo Hummus

This is a great alternative to the traditional legume-based hummus.

INGREDIENTS | SERVES 8

4 medium-sized beets, scrubbed, cooked, and cubed

¼ cup raw tahini paste

¼ cup lemon juice

1 small clove garlic, pressed

1. Place all ingredients in a food processor and pulse until smooth.

2. Chill and serve.

PER SERVING Calories: 63 | Fat: 4 g | Protein: 2 g | Sodium: 41 mg | Fiber: 2 g | Carbohydrate: 6 g

Tasty Baba Ganoush

*Eggplant is a great choice when looking for a complex carbohydrate source.
It has a slightly bitter taste, so be sure to cook it thoroughly.*

INGREDIENTS | SERVES 4

1 medium eggplant
2 tablespoons raw tahini paste
¼ cup lemon juice
4 cloves garlic
1 tablespoon olive oil

Eggplant Benefits

Eggplant skin contains a potent antioxidant and free radical scavenger called nasunin. This compound has been found to protect the fats that brain cells are composed of.

1. Bake eggplant for 30 minutes at 350°F, then cool.

2. Cut into 1" squares.

3. Place eggplant and all other ingredients into food processor and pulse until smooth.

4. Chill and serve.

PER SERVING Calories: 106 | Fat: 7.5 g | Protein: 2.5 g |
Sodium: 11 mg | Fiber: 4 g | Carbohydrate: 9 g

Paleo Chips

Most Paleolithic diet enthusiasts say they miss nacho chips the most. This is a close favorite and goes well with guacamole dip and salsa.

INGREDIENTS | **SERVES 3**

1 cup almond flour

½ cup flaxmeal

1 large egg

1 tablespoon garlic, minced

1 tablespoon organic, no-salt-added, tomato paste

1 jalapeño pepper, seeded and chopped

1 teaspoon chili powder

½ teaspoon onion powder

Complex Carbohydrates and the Paleolithic Diet

The most difficult transition from a Neolithic diet to a Paleolithic diet is in the letting go of high-carbohydrate snack foods such as chips and pretzels. Those comfort foods are associated with gatherings, parties, and celebrations. It will take a while to detox your body from such foods, but once you make the switch, you will not look back. The great way your body feels a couple of weeks into the plan more than makes up for the withdrawal from complex carbohydrates and refined sugar.

1. Preheat oven to 350°F.

2. Combine all ingredients into food processor and blend completely.

3. Spread evenly on a cookie sheet covered with parchment paper.

4. Bake for 10 minutes.

5. Remove from the oven and cut into squares.

6. Place back into the oven and continue baking for 5–10 minutes or until crunchy.

PER SERVING Calories: 239 | Fat: 8 g | Protein: 10 g | Sodium: 33 mg | Fiber: 8 g | Carbohydrate: 35 g

Roasted Parsnip Chips

Parsnips are a root vegetable related to the carrot. It has a sweet taste and has a lower glycemic load than potatoes.

INGREDIENTS | **SERVES 6**

Canola cooking spray
6 parsnips
3 tablespoons olive oil
⅛ teaspoon nutmeg
1 teaspoon cinnamon

1. Preheat oven to 400°F. Spray a cookie sheet with cooking spray.

2. Peel parsnips and cut at an angle to make long oval shapes.

3. In bowl, combine parsnips, olive oil, and spices. Mix well.

4. Spread parsnips out on cookie sheet in a single layer.

5. Cook 30 minutes. Remove from oven.

6. Turn on broiler.

7. Broil 5 minutes to make crispier chips.

PER SERVING Calories: 160 | Fat: 7 g | Protein: 1.5 g | Sodium: 14 mg | Fiber: 6.5 g | Carbohydrate: 24 g

Bison-Stuffed Zucchini

Bison meat is both low in fat and high in protein. It has a great taste that resembles beef, but with a little more flavor. This is sure to be a big hit at any party or holiday gathering.

INGREDIENTS | SERVES 6

3 large zucchini, halved

2 tablespoons coconut oil

1 cup onion, diced

1 cup cauliflower, chopped

1½ pounds bison meat, cubed

¼ teaspoon cayenne pepper

1 teaspoon oregano

1 (13.5-ounce) can no-salt-added diced tomatoes

1 (6-ounce) can organic, no-salt-added tomato paste

1 large egg

Bison: A Great Protein Choice

Bison meat is quite popular amongst Paleolithic diet enthusiasts. It is especially great for women due to its high iron content. Bison has more nutrients, pound for pound, than chicken, pork, or beef. It contains high levels of vitamins E, B_6, B_{12}, and such minerals as zinc, potassium, selenium, and copper.

1. Preheat oven to 400°F.

2. Scrape out seeds of zucchini and save in a mixing bowl.

3. Heat coconut oil in a skillet and sauté onion, cauliflower, and zucchini seeds until caramelized.

4. Add bison, cayenne pepper, and oregano to skillet and brown, approximately 8–10 minutes. Drain.

5. Add tomatoes and paste and stir to combine.

6. Combine bison mixture with vegetables and stir until blended.

7. Add egg, mix, and stuff each zucchini half forming large mound on top.

8. Place in large baking dish with a little water on the bottom and bake 40 minutes.

PER SERVING Calories: 214 | Fat: 7 g | Protein: 30 g | Sodium: 249 mg | Fiber: 3.5 g | Carbohydrate: 15 g

Rocking Salsa

This salsa is sure to be a winner at any party. Serve with Paleo Chips
(see this chapter) for a great appetizer before dinner.

INGREDIENTS | SERVES 2

½ cup chopped fresh cilantro

1½ cups chopped tomatoes

¼ cup sun-dried tomatoes

½ cup olive oil

2 teaspoons fresh-squeezed lime juice

1 teaspoon minced ginger

1½ teaspoons minced garlic

1 teaspoon minced jalapeño

Combine all ingredients in a food processor and pulse quickly to blend. Be careful not to over-pulse and completely liquefy this salsa. It should have a slight chunky texture.

PER SERVING Calories: 519 | Fat: 55 g | Protein: 2 g | Sodium: 146 mg | Fiber: 2 g | Carbohydrate: 9 g

Melon Salsa

*Salsa is always a delicious appetizer at parties. This sweet melon
salsa will add a new kick to the more traditional favorites.*

INGREDIENTS | SERVES 4

3 tomatoes, seeded and finely diced

½ honeydew melon, peeled and finely
diced

1 cantaloupe, peeled and finely diced

1 cup red onion, minced

½ jalapeño pepper, seeded and minced

½ cup chopped fresh cilantro

Juice of 1 large lime

1. In a large serving bowl, combine all ingredients and mix well.

2. Chill for 4 hours and serve.

PER SERVING Calories: 144 | Fat: 1 g | Protein: 4.5 g |
Sodium: 59 mg | Fiber: 4.5 g | Carbohydrate: 32 g

Melons

Melon has a very low sugar content. One
fruit serving of cantaloupe is half a melon.
This is a good choice when you're watching
calories or counting fruit servings per day.

Mango Creamsicle Sorbet

When the weather is hot and you're looking for a cold, refreshing treat, try this homemade sorbet recipe.

INGREDIENTS | SERVES 6

3 cups chopped peeled mangoes or fresh peaches

½ cup cold water

1 cup shredded coconut

2 tablespoons lemon juice

Sorbet

Try this recipe with other favorite fruits. If the sorbet does not seem sweet enough, add honey to the mixture next time. There is none added here because mango has a high sugar content on its own.

1. In a food processor or blender, combine mangoes and water; cover and process until smooth.

2. Add coconut and lemon juice; cover and process until smooth.

3. Transfer to container and freeze until solid, about 2 hours.

PER SERVING Calories: 80 | Fat: 4.5 g | Protein: 1.5 g | Sodium: 2.5 mg | Fiber: 3 g | Carbohydrate: 11 g

Tomato Juice

When you don't have time to eat your daily vegetable allowance, try whipping up this quick and easy tomato juice recipe to satisfy your daily needs.

INGREDIENTS | SERVES 2

1 (13.5-ounce) can unsalted, diced tomatoes

½ cup lemon juice

¼ cup lime juice

1 teaspoon pepper

⅛ teaspoon chili pepper

2 celery stalks, for garnish

1. Pour diced tomatoes into blender and blend until smooth.

2. Combine lemon juice, lime juice, pepper, and chili pepper and blend completely. Chill at least 1 hour.

3. Pour into glasses and garnish with celery.

PER SERVING Calories: 76 | Fat: 0.5 g | Protein: 3 g | Sodium: 374 mg | Fiber: 3 g | Carbohydrate: 17 g

Spiced Tea

This tea can be served hot or over ice. You can change the flavor quite easily with different tea bag flavors.

INGREDIENTS | SERVES 6

4 bags of herbal tea
1 teaspoon ground nutmeg
½ teaspoon ground cinnamon
¼ teaspoon ground cloves
6 cups boiling water

1. In a ceramic teapot, combine teabags and spices.

2. Pour boiling water into teapot. Steep for 5 minutes, then remove teabags.

PER SERVING Calories: 4 | Fat: 0 g | Protein: 0 g | Sodium: 2 g | Fiber: 0 g | Carbohydrate: 0 g

Vegetable Kebabs

*Serve these kebabs as an appetizer at parties so your guests
can easily handle the food without using cutlery.*

INGREDIENTS | SERVES 6

Wooden skewers

12 scallions

1 large red pepper

1 large yellow pepper

1 large green pepper

12 large button mushrooms

1 tablespoon olive oil

Freshly cracked black pepper, to taste

Soaking the Skewers

When using wooden skewers in cooking, always soak them in water for an hour before spearing the food items. Soaking the skewers allows you to place them on the grill for a time without them burning.

1. Cut standard wooden skewers in half for appetizer-size portions, then soak the skewers in water for a minimum of 1 hour.

2. Preheat grill or broiler.

3. Trim off the roots and dark green parts of the scallions. Dice the peppers into large pieces.

4. Thread the vegetables onto the skewers, and brush all sides of the vegetables with oil. Season with pepper.

5. Place the skewers on the grill or under the broiler, paying close attention as they cook, as they can easily burn. Cook until the vegetables are fork tender.

PER SERVING Calories: 38 | Fat: 2.5 g | Protein: 1 g | Sodium: 3.5 mg | Fiber: 2 g | Carbohydrate: 4 g

Groovy Guacamole

A favorite party appetizer with a major healthy punch.

INGREDIENTS | SERVES 4

2 large ripe avocados, coarsely chopped
1 small white onion, diced
1 tomato, unpeeled and diced
1 jalapeño pepper, thinly sliced
Juice of 1 lime

Gently combine all the ingredients in a serving bowl and serve as a salad or dip for whole-grain tortilla chips.

PER SERVING Calories: 136 | Fat: 11 g | Protein: 2 g | Sodium: 6.5 mg | Fiber: 5.5 g | Carbohydrate: 8 g

Avocados 101

Avocados are the main ingredient in guacamole. They may be high in fat, but it is the good anti-inflammatory, monounsaturated type. Avocados are also favorably high in fiber, potassium, many B vitamins, and vitamin E. Avocados darken easily when exposed to air, so it is best to save any leftovers with the pits and keep them in a tightly sealed container in the refrigerator. Use of lemon and lime juice in recipes will also keep discoloration at bay.

Mango Chutney

This fruity, cool chutney is a nice accompaniment to spicy dishes. To peel a ripe mango, you can slide a spoon, bottom side up, under the skin to remove it easily, without damaging the fruit.

INGREDIENTS | SERVES 8

3 mangoes
1 red onion
½ bunch fresh cilantro
1 teaspoon fresh lime juice
½ teaspoon freshly grated lime zest
Freshly cracked black pepper, to taste

Peel and dice the mangoes and onion. Chop the cilantro. Mix together all the ingredients in a medium-size bowl and adjust seasonings to taste.

PER SERVING Calories: 56 | Fat: 0 g | Protein: 1 g | Sodium: 1.5 mg | Fiber: 1.5 g | Carbohydrate: 13 g

Apple Chutney

Try this as a side for pork dishes instead of applesauce. It also is wonderful with hearty winter squash.

INGREDIENTS | **SERVES 4**

2 cups ice water

1 tablespoon fresh lemon juice

3 Granny Smith apples

1 shallot

3 sprigs fresh mint

1 tablespoon freshly grated lemon zest

¼ cup white raisins

½ teaspoon ground cinnamon

1. Combine the water and lemon juice in a large mixing bowl. Core and dice the unpeeled apples and place them in the lemon water.

2. Thinly slice the shallot and chop the mint.

3. Thoroughly drain the apples, then mix together all the ingredients in a medium-size bowl.

PER SERVING Calories: 80 | Fat: 0g | Protein: 0.5 g | Sodium: 2 mg | Fiber: 2.5 g | Carbohydrate: 21 g

CHAPTER 13

On the Barbecue

Grilled Lemon-and-Dill Swordfish Steaks

This recipe calls for preparation on the grill, but could easily be cooked in the oven using the broiler.

INGREDIENTS | SERVES 4

4 (4-ounce) swordfish steaks
1 tablespoon olive oil
1 lemon
4 dill sprigs

1. Coat swordfish steaks with light coating of olive oil.

2. Slice lemons into rings and place on top of swordfish steaks.

3. Place fresh dill sprig on each swordfish steak.

4. Grill over medium-high heat, about 10 minutes, depending on thickness of steak.

PER SERVING Calories: 134 | Fat: 6.5 g | Protein: 17 g | Sodium: 77 mg | Fiber: 0 g | Carbohydrate: 0 g

Salmon Skewers

Salmon has a wonderful omega profile being one of the highest sources of omega-3 fatty acid.

INGREDIENTS | SERVES 4

8 ounces salmon fillet

1 red onion, cut into wedges

2 red bell peppers, cut into 2" squares

12 mushrooms

12 cherry tomatoes

Wild-Caught Versus Farm-Raised Salmon

Salmon is one of the best sources of omega-3 fatty acids, but be sure to purchase wild-caught salmon. Farm-raised salmon is not exposed to the colder water, and therefore their fat reserves are not as robust as wild salmon.

1. Cut salmon into cubes.

2. Thread all ingredients on metal skewers, alternating vegetables and meat.

3. Grill over medium-high heat until vegetables are soft and salmon is light pink, about 10 minutes, depending on thickness of salmon steak.

PER SERVING Calories: 107 | Fat: 3.5 g | Protein: 15 g | Sodium: 235 mg | Fiber: 2.5 g | Carbohydrate: 6.5 g

Tilapia with Tomato and Dill

Tilapia is a very low fat fish choice with a light flavor. It cooks quickly and absorbs flavors from spices quite nicely.

INGREDIENTS | **SERVES 6**

6 tilapia filets
2 large beefsteak tomatoes, sliced
6 rosemary sprigs

1. Place each tilapia filet on a square of aluminum foil.

2. Cover each filet with 2–3 slices of tomato and a sprig of rosemary.

3. Fold and seal foil over each filet and grill over medium heat for 6 to 8 minutes, or until fish flakes easily.

PER SERVING Calories: 122 | Fat: 2.5 g | Protein: 23 g | Sodium: 53 mg | Fiber: 0.5 g | Carbohydrate: 2.5 g

Spicy Grilled Flank Steak

Flank steak is one of the leanest steak cuts. It is usually the best and safest choice of steak to order when going out to dinner, as well.

INGREDIENTS | SERVES 4

2 tablespoons raw honey

1 teaspoon cinnamon

1 teaspoon chili powder

½ teaspoon salt-free lemon pepper seasoning

1½ pounds lean flank steak

½ cup sliced green onions

1. Combine honey, cinnamon, chili powder, and lemon-pepper seasoning in a small bowl.

2. Grill flank steak over medium-high heat covered for 6 minutes on each side. Baste often with honey mixture.

3. Serve sprinkled with green onions as garnish.

PER SERVING Calories: 368 | Fat: 12 g | Protein: 52 g | Sodium: 113 mg | Fiber: 0.5 g | Carbohydrate: 9.5 g

Flank Steak and Good Fat

Flank steak is a terrific choice when you want a lower-fat version of red meat. This steak usually contains less than 13 grams of fat per serving, while some other more fatty cuts have about 20 grams of fat per serving.

Lemon-Thyme Grilled Swordfish

Thyme is a useful spice that adds flavor without overpowering a dish, and it blends well with other spices.

INGREDIENTS | SERVES 4

4 (4-ounce) swordfish steaks
1 cup water
3 tablespoons fresh lemon juice
1 bay leaf
1 teaspoon dried thyme, crushed

1. Preheat barbecue grill to 350°F.

2. Place the fish in aluminum foil wrapping.

3. Pour the water and lemon juice over fish. Add bay leaf.

4. Sprinkle the thyme over the fish and wrap the foil closed.

5. Cook for 10 minutes or until the fish flakes easily when tested with a fork and is opaque all the way through.

PER SERVING Calories: 107 | Fat: 3.5 g | Protein: 17 g | Sodium: 77 mg | Fiber: 0 g | Carbohydrate: 1 g

Shrimp Skewers

These skewers are easy to make and can be served as a main dish or an appetizer. They are fantastic at parties or holiday celebrations.

INGREDIENTS | SERVES 4

1½ pounds large shrimp, peeled and deveined

Juice of ½ lime

1 teaspoon ground black pepper

1 medium zucchini, sliced in 1" pieces

1 medium summer squash, sliced in 1" pieces

1 large red bell pepper, sliced in 2" × 2" pieces

1 large green bell pepper, sliced in 2" × 2" pieces

4 cloves garlic, finely minced

2 tablespoons olive oil

1. Soak 8 wooden skewers in water for at least 30 minutes.

2. In a large bowl, drizzle shrimp with lime juice and season with pepper. Set aside for 5 minutes.

3. Add vegetables, garlic, and olive oil to the shrimp and toss to coat.

4. Alternate vegetables and shrimp on skewers.

5. Grill over medium heat for 5 minutes or until shrimp turns pink, then turn skewers to cook other side an additional 5 minutes.

PER SERVING Calories: 209 | Fat: 9.5 g | Protein: 26 g | Sodium: 190 mg | Fiber: 0.5 g | Carbohydrate: 4.5 g

Shrimp and Omega-3

Shrimp is a good source of omega-3 fatty acids. This terrific shellfish is naturally low in fat and high in protein. If you have high cholesterol, you might want to watch your intake. They do have higher levels than other protein sources.

Grilled Salmon

Salmon is a traditional barbecue item and a staple in the Paleolithic diet. This omega-3 heavyweight is sure to please everyone at the family barbecue.

INGREDIENTS | SERVES 4

2 pounds salmon fillets

½ cup olive oil

½ cup lemon juice

4 green onions, thinly sliced

3 tablespoons minced fresh parsley

2 teaspoons minced fresh rosemary

⅛ teaspoon pepper

Olive Oil and Grilling

Although there are many oils to choose from, most recipes in this book use olive oil. Olive oil has a high heat tolerance and low smoke value. This makes it ideal for cooking, particularly on the grill.

1. Place salmon in shallow dish.

2. Combine remaining ingredients in a medium bowl and mix well. Set aside ¼ cup for basting and pour the rest over the salmon.

3. Cover and refrigerate salmon for 30 minutes.

4. Grill salmon over medium heat, skin side down, for 15–20 minutes. Baste with marinade often.

PER SERVING Calories: 490 | Fat: 38 g | Protein: 34 g | Sodium: 78 mg | Fiber: 0 g | Carbohydrate: 3 g

Jalapeño Steak

When you want a little kick of flavor instead of the more traditional steak meals, give this recipe a shot. Jalapeños and lime juice give this meal a cultural feel.

INGREDIENTS | SERVES 6

4 jalapeño peppers, stemmed and roughly chopped

4 cloves garlic, peeled

1½ teaspoons cracked black pepper

1 tablespoon sea salt

¼ cup lime juice

1 tablespoon dried oregano

1½ pounds top sirloin steak

1. Combine jalapeños, garlic, pepper, sea salt, lime juice, and oregano in a blender. Blend until smooth.

2. Place steak in a shallow pan and pour marinade over it. Marinate for 8 hours.

3. Drain and discard marinade. Grill steak over high heat for 5 minutes per side, or to desired doneness.

PER SERVING Calories: 229 | Fat: 8 g | Protein: 35 g | Sodium: 1,238 mg | Fiber: 0 g | Carbohydrate: 2 g

Sea Salt

Strict Paleolithic diet followers would not use salt in any form, but looser followers add organic sea salt to recipes where salt is desired. Sea salt is often used for steaks and other grilled meats.

BBQ Chicken

This mouthwatering chicken will become a staple in your home regardless of the season.

INGREDIENTS | SERVES 4

3 tablespoons olive oil

1½ cups apple cider vinegar

½ cup raw honey

Juice of 1 lemon

¼ teaspoon ground black pepper

5 fresh sage sprigs

2 pounds bone-in chicken breasts

Cage-Free and Barn-Roaming

Cage-free and barn-roaming chickens are the best chickens to purchase. Chickens that are given feedlot grains derived from corn have a less attractive fat profile. Commercial farms tend to use antibiotics and growth hormones. All of these products eventually leach into our bodies where they can magnify over time.

1. In a small bowl combine olive oil, vinegar, honey, lemon juice, pepper, and sage.

2. Place chicken breasts on hot grill and baste with sauce.

3. Cook for 45–60 minutes, turning every 10–15 minutes. Baste with sauce after each turning.

PER SERVING Calories: 389 | Fat: 12 g | Protein: 35 g | Sodium: 7 mg | Fiber: 0 g | Carbohydrate: 36 g

Grilled Trout

Cooking the fish inside the foil packets keeps it tender and moist.

INGREDIENTS | SERVES 2

2 whole trout, heads removed, cleaned and butterflied

1 teaspoon ground black pepper

2 cloves garlic, minced

½ teaspoon chopped fresh rosemary

1 teaspoon chopped fresh parsley

6 sprigs fresh rosemary

1 lemon, halved; one half thinly sliced

Oily Fishes

There are many fishes that are good sources of beneficial fatty acids. These fish include trout, sardines, swordfish, whitebait, fresh tuna, anchovies, eel, kipper, mackerel, carp, bloater, smelt, and bluefish. The more variety of fish that you try, the better fatty acid profile you will compile.

1. Place each trout on a square piece of aluminum.

2. Season both sides of trout with pepper, garlic, chopped rosemary, and parsley.

3. Fold fish closed and top with rosemary sprigs and a few slices of lemon.

4. Squeeze the lemon half over each fish.

5. Wrap each fish securely inside the sheet of aluminum foil.

6. Grill packets over medium-high heat for 7 minutes on each side or until fish is flaky.

PER SERVING Calories: 176 | Fat: 8 g | Protein: 25 g | Sodium: 62 mg | Fiber: 0 g | Carbohydrate: 0 g

Grilled Pineapple

Pineapple has such a profound flavor, and grilling just intensifies it. The addition of some raw honey will make this a really special treat at any barbecue or party.

INGREDIENTS | SERVES 6

Nonstick cooking spray

1 fresh pineapple, cored, peeled, and cut into 1" rings

¼ cup raw honey

2 tablespoons chopped macadamia nuts

1. Coat grill rack with nonstick cooking spray before starting the grill.

2. Grill pineapple over medium heat for 5 minutes.

3. Turn pineapple over and grill 5 more minutes.

4. Brush with honey and sprinkle with macadamia nuts.

PER SERVING Calories: 102 | Fat: 2 g | Protein: 1 g | Sodium: 1.5 mg | Fiber: 1 g | Carbohydrate: 22 g

Rich in Omega-3

Super Omega Salmon Cakes

These salmon cakes are a great party appetizer. Even non-Paleolithic dieters will rave about them.

INGREDIENTS | SERVES 10

3 pounds salmon, finely diced

⅔ cup egg white

1 teaspoon dried dill

¼ teaspoon ground ginger

¼ teaspoon cayenne pepper

¼ cup black pepper

¼ cup fresh squeezed lemon juice

¼ cup grapeseed oil

¼ cup flaxseed flour

1 cup almond meal

Super Omega

The more omega-3 fatty acid you ingest, the better chance you will have at fighting silent inflammation. It is also proven to significantly reduce your recovery time from workouts or endurance races. The more omega-3, the better for optimum health all around.

1. Preheat broiler.

2. Mix salmon, egg white, dill, ginger, cayenne, black pepper, lemon juice, oil, and flaxseed flour together in a large bowl.

3. Form about 20 small patties from the mixture.

4. Pour almond meal into a shallow dish.

5. Dredge patties in almond meal and place on an ungreased cookie sheet.

6. Broil each side for 4 minutes.

PER SERVING Calories: 221 | Fat: 9 g | Protein: 24 g | Sodium: 72 mg | Fiber: 2 g | Carbohydrate: 13 g

Salmon in Parchment with Baby Brussels Sprouts

Cooking the salmon in parchment paper works to keep the fish from drying out, a common problem when cooking fish in the oven. The paper also helps to contain flavors so they are not cooked off.

INGREDIENTS | SERVES 2

2 (4- to 5-ounce) salmon fillets or steaks

2 tablespoons frozen petite Brussels sprouts

2 cloves garlic, crushed

2 dashes lemon juice

1 tablespoon olive oil

1. Preheat oven to 425°F.

2. Place each piece of salmon on a large (12") circle of parchment paper.

3. Cover each salmon piece with a spoonful of Brussels sprouts, a clove of crushed garlic, a squeeze of lemon juice, and a drizzle of olive oil.

4. Fold the paper over into a packet and seal the edges by crimping and folding like a pastry. Place on a baking sheet.

5. Bake for 15 minutes, or until fish flakes easily with a fork.

PER SERVING Calories: 189 | Fat: 12 g | Protein: 17 g | Sodium: 39 mg | Fiber: 0.5 g | Carbohydrate: 1.5 g

Flaxseed Smoothie

This quick treat is a great snack with the powerful punch of high omega-3 fatty acids. Strawberries contain high antioxidant levels to make this smoothie a perfect and refreshing snack on a hot afternoon.

INGREDIENTS | **SERVES 1**

½ frozen peeled banana, cut into slices

1 cup frozen strawberries

2 tablespoons flaxseed meal

1 cup vanilla coconut, almond, or hazelnut milk

Place all ingredients in blender. Purée until smooth.

PER SERVING Calories: 410 | Fat: 14 g | Protein: 14 g | Sodium: 146 mg | Fiber: 16 g | Carbohydrate: 64 g

Flaxseed

Flax is a great way to introduce more omega-3 fatty acids into your diet. These little powerhouses are small, easily transported, and virtually tasteless. They can be added easily into any smoothie or salad for a little anti-inflammatory benefit.

Citrus-Baked Snapper

Snapper is a tasty fish that absorbs the flavors in the recipe quite nicely.

INGREDIENTS | SERVES 4

1 (3-pound) whole red snapper, cleaned and scaled

3½ tablespoons grated fresh gingerroot

3 green onions, chopped

1 tomato, seeded and diced

¼ cup fresh squeezed orange juice

¼ cup fresh squeezed lime juice

¼ cup fresh squeezed lemon juice

3 thin slices lime

3 thin slices lemon

Snapper and Omega-3

Snapper is not the fish that comes to mind when you're thinking about omega-3, but this cold water fish does have some beneficial DHA fatty acid packed inside. Those with elevated blood triglycerides will benefit greatly from even small amounts of EPA and DHA.

1. Preheat the oven to 350°F.

2. Make three slashes across each side of the fish using a sharp knife. This will keep the fish from curling as it cooks.

3. Place the fish in a shallow baking dish or roasting pan.

4. Cover each side of fish with ginger, green onions, and tomatoes.

5. Combine juices and drizzle over snapper.

6. Place lime and lemon slices on top of fish.

7. Cover with aluminum foil and bake until the flesh is opaque and can be flaked with a fork, about 20 minutes.

PER SERVING Calories: 271 | Fat: 3.5 g | Protein: 53 g | Sodium: 166 mg | Fiber: 0.5 g | Carbohydrate: 4 g

Salmon with Leeks

Salmon and leeks complement each other well. The leeks have a strong taste to balance out the flavor of the salmon. This recipe is a nice combination of two great tastes.

INGREDIENTS | SERVES 4

4 leeks
2 tablespoons coconut butter
1 tablespoon raw honey
3 carrots, cut into matchsticks
2 pounds salmon fillets
2 teaspoons olive oil
1 teaspoon ground black pepper

Leeks Are a Healthy Choice

Not only are leeks high in fiber, but they also contain folic acid, calcium, potassium, and vitamin C. Leeks are quite antiseptic and have been found to have anti-arthritic properties.

1. Preheat oven to 425°F.

2. Trim leeks and discard root end and outer leaves. Cut lengthwise.

3. Melt coconut butter in a large skillet over medium-high heat, add leeks, and cook until soft, about 5 minutes.

4. Drizzle the leeks with honey and cook until they turn brown, 15–20 minutes.

5. Stir in carrots and cook until tender, about 10 minutes.

6. Line a baking sheet with foil and spray with cooking spray. Place salmon on baking sheet. Brush salmon with olive oil and sprinkle with black pepper.

7. Roast the salmon in oven until flesh is pink and flaky. Serve salmon topped with leek and carrot mixture.

PER SERVING Calories: 423 | Fat: 19 g | Protein: 37 g | Sodium: 160 mg | Fiber: 4.5 g | Carbohydrate: 27 g

Fried Sardines

There are not many fried items in a Paleolithic diet, because most fried dishes are made with flour. This is a healthier alternative to traditional frying. The alcohol in the wine is mostly cooked off, so you will not have to worry about the alcohol either.

INGREDIENTS | SERVES 6

1 cup almond flour
2 pounds skinless, boneless, no-salt-added sardines
¾ cup plus 1 tablespoon olive oil
2 cloves garlic, chopped
1 cup white wine
1 cup apple cider vinegar
½ cup chopped mint leaves

Mercury in Fish

Sardines are a great source of omega-3, but lack the dangerous mercury worries that other cold-water fish higher up on the food chain have. On lower level fish, mercury is not amplified and therefore does not pose as much of a risk for humans.

1. Pour almond flour into a shallow dish.

2. Roll sardines in almond flour.

3. Heat ¾ cup olive oil in a large skillet over medium-high heat.

4. When the oil is hot, fry the sardines until brown and crispy, approximately 5 minutes. Drain on paper towels and keep warm.

5. In another skillet over medium heat, warm garlic in remaining olive oil. Cook for 1 minute.

6. Add the wine and vinegar. Simmer mixture, stirring occasionally, until the liquid has reduced by half, about 15 minutes.

7. Pour the sauce over the sardines, and sprinkle with fresh mint.

PER SERVING Calories: 318 | Fat: 14 g | Protein: 31 g | Sodium: 575 mg | Fiber: 2.5 g | Carbohydrate: 18 g

Grilled Salmon

Grilling salmon is a nice way to get maximum flavor while cooking. The marinade in this recipe doubles as a basting sauce to really seal in the flavor.

INGREDIENTS | SERVES 4

2 pounds salmon fillets
½ cup vegetable oil
½ cup lemon juice
4 green onions, thinly sliced
3 tablespoons minced fresh parsley
1½ teaspoons minced fresh rosemary
⅛ teaspoon pepper

1. Place salmon in shallow dish.

2. In a medium bowl, combine remaining ingredients and mix well. Set aside ¼ cup for basting; pour the rest over the salmon.

3. Cover and refrigerate for 30 minutes. Drain, discarding marinade.

4. Grill salmon over medium heat, skin side down, for 15–20 minutes or until fish flakes easily with a fork. Baste occasionally with reserved marinade.

PER SERVING Calories: 492 | Fat: 39 g | Protein: 34 g | Sodium: 75 mg | Fiber: 0.5 g | Carbohydrate: 0.5 g

Curried Scrambled Eggs

Eggs from barn-roaming and cage-free chickens are naturally high in omega-3.

INGREDIENTS | SERVES 1

2 large omega-3, cage-free eggs

1 teaspoon water

1 teaspoon finely chopped chives

⅛ teaspoon curry powder

1 teaspoon olive oil

Omega-3 Eggs

Omega-3 eggs are eggs that are from chickens that were fed a diet high in omega-3 fatty acids. The more fatty acids the chickens eat, the more that is passed on to you. This is a great way to get EFAs without eating fish all the time.

1. In a small bowl, beat eggs, water, chives, and curry powder.

2. Heat oil in a medium frying pan over medium heat.

3. Scramble eggs for 5 minutes or until set.

PER SERVING Calories: 190 | Fat: 15 g | Protein: 12 g | Sodium: 126 mg | Fiber: 0 g | Carbohydrate: 2 g

Mackerel with Tomato and Cucumber Salad

According to the USDA Nutrient Database, mackerel contains 2.3 grams of omega-3 for every 100 grams of fish. That makes mackerel the highest EFA-containing fish.

INGREDIENTS | SERVES 4

15 ounces mackerel fillets, drained
1 clove garlic, crushed
1½ tablespoons flaxseed oil
1 tablespoon chopped fresh basil
½ teaspoon ground black pepper
10 cherry tomatoes, halved
½ cucumber, peeled and diced
1 small onion, chopped
2 cups mixed lettuce greens

1. Place mackerel in a medium bowl with garlic and flaxseed oil.

2. Add basil and pepper to mackerel mixture and sauté over medium heat for 5–8 minutes each side, or until brown.

3. Cut cooked mackerel into bite-size pieces and add to bowl.

4. Stir in tomatoes, cucumber, onion, lettuce and serve.

PER SERVING Calories: 235 | Fat: 16 g | Protein: 16 g | Sodium: 82 mg | Fiber: 1 g | Carbohydrate: 3.5 g

Pecan-Crusted Salmon

Sushi-grade salmon is very high quality and it is safe to eat mostly raw. Obtain this quality fish from a fish company that specializes in high-end fish to ensure quality.

INGREDIENTS | SERVES 4

1 cup crushed pecans
4 (4-ounce) sushi-grade salmon filets
2 tablespoons coconut oil

1. Spread crushed pecans on a flat surface.

2. Place salmon on pecans and coat all sides.

3. Preheat frying pan over high heat and add coconut oil to coat pan.

4. Flash cook salmon quickly on each side, 2–3 minutes.

PER SERVING Calories: 370 | Fat: 32 g | Protein: 19 g | Sodium: 38 mg | Fiber: 3 g | Carbohydrate: 4 g

Haddock Fish Cakes

This version of a familiar fish cake has the fresh flavor of haddock.
Serve this with a spicy sauce or a fresh spritz of lemon.

INGREDIENTS | SERVES 6

1 pound haddock

2 leeks

1 red pepper

2 egg whites

Freshly cracked black pepper, to taste

1 tablespoon olive oil

1. Finely shred the raw fish with a fork. Dice the leeks and red pepper. Combine all the ingredients except the oil in a medium-size bowl; mix well. Form the mixture into small oval patties.

2. Heat the oil in a medium-size sauté pan. Place the cakes in the pan and loosely cover with the lid; sauté the cakes for 4–6 minutes on each side. Drain on a rack covered with paper towels; serve immediately.

PER SERVING Calories: 97 | Fat: 3 g | Protein: 13 g | Sodium: 67 mg | Fiber: 1 g | Carbohydrate: 5 g

Fresh Tuna with Sweet Lemon Leek Salsa

The tuna can be prepared the night before, refrigerated, then either reheated or served at room temperature.

INGREDIENTS | **SERVES 6**

Tuna

1½ pounds fresh tuna steaks (cut into 4-ounce portions)

¼–½ teaspoon extra-virgin olive oil

Freshly cracked black pepper, to taste

Salsa

1 teaspoon extra-virgin olive oil

3 fresh leeks (light green and white parts only), thinly sliced

1 tablespoon fresh lemon juice

1 tablespoon honey

Tuna Packs a Punch

Tuna is truly a nutrient-dense food. This omega-3 fatty acid–rich food has anti-inflammation written all over it with heaps of other valuable disease-fighting nutrients as well. Health authorities are urging consumers to gobble up fish two times per week to reap the significant health benefits.

1. Preheat grill to medium-high temperature.

2. Brush each portion of the tuna with the oil and drain on a rack. Season the tuna with pepper, then place the tuna on the grill; cook for 3 minutes. Shift the tuna steaks on the grill to form an X grill pattern; cook 3 more minutes.

3. Turn the steaks over and grill 3 more minutes, then change position again to create an X grill pattern. Cook to desired doneness.

4. For the salsa: Heat the oil in a medium-size sauté pan on medium heat, then add the leeks. When the leeks are wilted, add the lemon juice and honey. Plate each tuna portion with a spoonful of salsa.

PER SERVING Calories: 171 | Fat: 5.5 g | Protein: 21 g | Sodium: 43 mg | Fiber: 1 g | Carbohydrate: 9.5 g

Lime-Poached Flounder

Lime brings out the delicate flavor of the fish and complements the zip of the cilantro.

INGREDIENTS | **SERVES 6**

¾ cup leek, sliced

¼ cup cilantro, leaves separated from stems

1½ pounds flounder fillets

1¾ cups fish stock

2 tablespoons fresh lime juice

½ teaspoon fresh lime zest

¼ teaspoon black pepper, ground

1 cup yellow onion, shredded

⅔ cup carrots, shredded

⅔ cup celery, shredded

2 tablespoons extra-virgin olive oil

Using Frozen Fish

Don't fret if you do not have fresh fish available in your area. Using a quality fish frozen at sea is perfectly fine. In fact, sometimes the frozen fish is fresher than the fresh!

1. Place the leek slices and cilantro stems (reserve the leaves) in a large skillet, then lay the flounder on top.

2. Add the stock, lime juice, lime zest, and pepper. Bring to simmer, cover, and cook for 7–10 minutes, until the flounder is thoroughly cooked. Remove from heat. Strain off and discard the liquid.

3. To serve, lay the shredded onions, carrots, and celery in separate strips on serving plates. Top with flounder, drizzle with the extra-virgin olive oil, and sprinkle with the reserved cilantro leaves.

PER SERVING Calories: 150 | Fat: 6 g | Protein: 18 g | Sodium: 218 mg | Fiber: 1 g | Carbohydrate: 3.5 g

Grilled Halibut Herb Salad

*If you don't care for oranges, or don't have any fresh ones handy,
use drained capers to garnish the entrée salad instead.*

INGREDIENTS | SERVES 2

2 (6-ounce) halibut fillets

4 teaspoons orange juice

3 tablespoons olive oil

¼ teaspoon lemon pepper

¼ teaspoon garlic powder

¼ teaspoon sweet Hungarian paprika

2 cups romaine lettuce, torn

¼ cup flat-leaf parsley, chopped

1 tablespoon fresh basil, chopped

1 tablespoon fresh chives, sliced

2 orange slices

1. Place a large grill pan over medium-high heat. Sprinkle each fillet side with 1 teaspoon of orange juice and lightly rub it in. Brush both sides of each fillet with oil. Sprinkle each side with a little lemon pepper, garlic powder, and paprika.

2. Add fillets to hot grill pan and cook for 5 minutes on each side. Remove fillets from pan as soon as they are cooked and place on a plate. Let fillets rest for 3 minutes, then slice each one widthwise.

3. Combine romaine, parsley, basil, and chives in a large salad bowl. Toss to mix. Split salad between two plates. Top each salad with a sliced fillet. Squeeze an orange slice over each salad, garnish with slice, and serve.

PER SERVING Calories: 317 | Fat: 23 g | Protein: 24 g | Sodium: 179 mg | Fiber: 2 g | Carbohydrate: 5 g

CHAPTER 15

Avocado Favorites

Avocado Chicken Salad

This recipe is a great party salad. You can serve it in lettuce cups for a meal or in small cups with spoons as an appetizer.

INGREDIENTS | SERVES 3

3 avocados, pitted and peeled

2 boneless, skinless chicken breasts, cooked and shredded

½ red onion, chopped

1 large tomato, chopped

¼ cup chopped cilantro

Juice of 1 large lime

1. In a medium bowl, mash avocados. Add chicken and mix well.

2. Add onion, tomato, cilantro, and lime juice to the avocado and chicken mixture. Mix well and serve.

PER SERVING Calories: 340 | Fat: 23 g | Protein: 26 g | Sodium: 10 mg | Fiber: 10 g | Carbohydrate: 13 g

Asparagus and Avocado Lettuce Wraps

This recipe is a great side dish for any main course. Or add protein to make a complete meal.

INGREDIENTS | SERVES 4

24 asparagus spears
1 ripe avocado, pitted and peeled
1 tablespoon fresh-squeezed lime juice
1 clove garlic, minced
2 cups chopped tomato
2 tablespoons chopped red onion
3–4 whole romaine lettuce leaves
⅓ cup fresh cilantro leaves, chopped

Health Benefits of Asparagus

Asparagus is an often undervalued vegetable in the kitchen. This healthy stalk weighs in at a healthy 60 percent RDA of folic acid. Additionally, it is high in vitamins A, B_6, and C, as well as potassium and folic acid. Asparagus is a great vegetable to eat if you're trying to lose weight. It has a diuretic effect and helps you to release excess water from the body.

1. In a medium-sized saucepan over high heat, bring 2" water to a boil.

2. Place the asparagus in a steamer basket, cover, and steam until just tender. Be careful not to overcook. The asparagus should still have a bit of crunch after about 5 minutes of steaming.

3. Remove asparagus and immediately rinse in cold water. Drain thoroughly.

4. In a small bowl, mash the avocado, lime juice, and garlic into a coarse purée.

5. In another bowl stir together the tomatoes and onions.

6. Lay the lettuce leaves flat and spread avocado mixture equally among the lettuce leaves then add tomato and onion mixture.

7. Top with a dash of fresh cilantro leaves.

8. Fold in both sides and the bottom of each lettuce leaf.

PER SERVING Calories: 75 | Fat: 5.5 g | Protein: 2.5 g | Sodium: 4.5 mg | Fiber: 4.5 g | Carbohydrate: 6.5 g

Guacamole

Guacamole has the perfect balance of fat, carbohydrates, and protein to fill you up and balance your hormone levels.

INGREDIENTS | SERVES 6

3 very ripe avocados, pitted and peeled

Juice of 2 limes

½ cup diced red onion

1 cup diced plum tomatoes

¼ cup diced jalapeño peppers

½ cup chopped fresh cilantro

1. Mash avocados in a medium bowl.

2. Add all other ingredients to avocado, mix and serve.

PER SERVING Calories: 131 | Fat: 11 g | Protein: 2 g | Sodium: 8 mg | Fiber: 6 g | Carbohydrate: 8 g

Medicinal Properties of Cilantro

Cilantro, also called coriander, is an herb that has been used for many medicinal purposes. It is known to aid in digestive disorders, can help settle upset stomach, reduces minor swelling, and helps to promote healthy liver function.

Avocado-Eggplant Spread

*Eggplant and avocado together make a filling and healthy dip. Add
this recipe to salads or use as dip with cut vegetables.*

INGREDIENTS | SERVES 4

2 medium eggplants, skinned and
roasted

¼ cup tahini

2 cloves of garlic, minced

2 tablespoons fresh lime juice

½ teaspoon ground black pepper

½ teaspoon cumin

1 avocado, pitted, peeled, and cubed

Combine all ingredients in a food processor and pulse
until desired consistency is reached.

PER SERVING Calories: 202 | Fat: 13 g | Protein: 6 g |
Sodium: 18 mg | Fiber: 11 g | Carbohydrate: 21 g

Avocado Smoothie

This quick blended smoothie is a sweet treat when you're looking for something refreshing that resembles a milkshake.

INGREDIENTS | **SERVES 1**

1 ripe avocado, pitted and peeled

1 cup coconut milk

½ cup almond milk

3 tablespoons raw honey

3–4 ice cubes

In a blender combine all ingredients until smooth. Serve chilled.

PER SERVING Calories: 774 | Fat: 53 g | Protein: 10 g | Sodium: 98 mg | Fiber: 14 g | Carbohydrate: 80 g

Avocado Milkshakes

In the Philippines, Brazil, Indonesia, Vietnam, and south India, avocados are often used in milkshakes. If you are craving a delicious chocolate treat try this recipe with added cacao nibs.

Fried Avocado

This recipe is high in fat, but mostly in the omega-3 fatty acid side. If you want to watch your fat intake, cut the recipe in half and serve as a side dish with a main protein source.

INGREDIENTS | **SERVES 2**

1–2 cups olive oil for frying
1 cup almond meal
1 pinch ground cumin
1 egg, beaten
1 avocado, peeled, pitted, and sliced

1. Heat oil in a large heavy skillet or deep-fryer to 365°F.

2. In a small bowl, mix together the almond meal and cumin.

3. Place the beaten egg in a shallow dish.

4. Dip avocado slices in beaten egg, and then in the almond meal mixture.

5. Drop avocado into oil and fry until golden brown on both sides, approximately 5 minutes per side.

PER SERVING Calories: 617 | Fat: 43 g | Protein: 9.5 g | Sodium: 59 mg | Fiber: 9.5 g | Carbohydrate: 54 g

Avocado Salad

This salad is a refreshing choice on a hot summer day when you want something cold and satisfying.

INGREDIENTS | **SERVES 4**

2 avocados, peeled, pitted, and diced

1 small sweet onion, chopped

1 medium red bell pepper, chopped

1 large ripe tomato, chopped

¼ cup chopped fresh cilantro

Juice of ½ lime

1. In a medium bowl, combine all ingredients.

2. Mix well and chill for at least 2 hours before serving.

PER SERVING Calories: 159 | Fat: 11 g | Protein: 3 g | Sodium: 14 mg | Fiber: 7 g | Carbohydrate: 16 g

Red Versus Green Peppers

Although green and red peppers are both healthy choices, red peppers contain a very high amount of vitamins A and C. One medium red pepper can contribute a whopping 75 percent of vitamin A and 253 percent of vitamin C, compared with 9 percent vitamin A and 159 percent vitamin C per medium green pepper.

Avocado-Watermelon Salad

This salad is packed with flavor. The watermelon adds a sweet touch to an otherwise plain salad.

INGREDIENTS | SERVES 4

2 large avocados, pitted, peeled, and diced

4 cups cubed watermelon

4 cups fresh baby spinach leaves

½ cup walnut oil

Juice of 1 lime

½ teaspoon sweet paprika

In a medium bowl, combine all ingredients. Mix well and serve.

PER SERVING Calories: 414 | Fat: 40 g | Protein: 4 g | Sodium: 31 mg | Fiber: 6 g | Carbohydrate: 20 g

Exotic Fruit Guacamole

Papaya and mango add an exotic twist to a traditional dish. The mix of sour and sweet will make your taste buds crave more of this delicious appetizer recipe.

INGREDIENTS | SERVES 4

1 medium papaya, cubed

1 medium mango, cubed

1 medium ripe avocado, pitted, peeled, and diced

1 tablespoon lime juice

2 cups diced, seeded tomato

¼ cup diced onion

2 tablespoons minced fresh cilantro

1 teaspoon seeded, finely chopped jalapeño pepper

1 garlic clove, minced

In a medium bowl, combine all ingredients. Mix well and serve.

PER SERVING Calories: 120 | Fat: 6 g | Protein: 2.5 g | Sodium: 13 mg | Fiber: 5 g | Carbohydrate: 18 g

Papaya, "Fruit of the Angels"

The exotic and sweet papaya contains over 300 percent of your daily vitamin C. It is a rich source of potassium and vitamins A, E, and K. A papaya also contains almost 30 percent of the recommended daily intake of folate. Folate is particularly good for pregnant women.

Avocado-Orange Lettuce Wraps

These light and delicious wraps taste like summer on a plate.

INGREDIENTS | SERVES 4

4 large romaine lettuce leaves

1 large navel orange, peeled and cut into ¼" thick slices

2 large avocados, pitted, peeled, and sliced

1 (5-ounce) package alfalfa sprouts

Juice of 1 lemon

1. Arrange lettuce leaves on 4 plates.

2. Place even numbers of orange slices on top of lettuce leaves.

3. Stack avocado slices and sprouts on top of each leaf.

4. Squeeze lemon juice over the top of each pile.

5. Fold leaf, place toothpick through wrap to hold in place, and serve.

PER SERVING Calories: 148 | Fat: 11 g | Protein: 3 g | Sodium: 8 g | Fiber: 7 g | Carbohydrate: 12 g

Crisp Avocado Salad

This recipe works well as a side dish to spicy Southwest or Mexican entrées.

INGREDIENTS | SERVES 4

3 cups iceberg lettuce, shredded

2 cups avocado, chopped

½ cup red onion, sliced

1 (3-ounce) can black olives, sliced

1 tablespoon lime juice

2 tablespoons toasted pine nuts

Toss lettuce, avocado, onion, and olives together in a large salad bowl. Sprinkle salad with lime juice. Toss well to coat. Sprinkle with pine nuts and serve.

PER SERVING Calories: 189 | Fat: 17 g | Protein: 3 g | Sodium: 72 mg | Fiber: 6 g | Carbohydrate: 10 g

Salads, Dressings, and Sauces

Recipes (continued)

Apple Coleslaw

This coleslaw recipe is a refreshing and sweet alternative to the traditional coleslaw with mayonnaise. Additionally, the sesame seeds give it a nice, nutty flavor.

INGREDIENTS | SERVES 4

2 cups packaged coleslaw mix

1 unpeeled tart apple, chopped

½ cup chopped celery

½ cup chopped green pepper

¼ cup flaxseed oil

2 tablespoons lemon juice

1 teaspoon sesame seeds

1. In a bowl combine the coleslaw mix, apple, celery, and green pepper.

2. In a small bowl, whisk remaining ingredients. Pour over coleslaw and toss to coat.

PER SERVING Calories: 158 | Fat: 14 g | Protein: 1 g | Sodium: 20 mg | Fiber: 2.5 g | Carbohydrate: 8.5 g

Seeds Versus Nuts

Nuts have a higher omega-6 to omega-3 ratio. Seeds, on the other hand, have a much different profile. Seeds have much lower saturated fat content and are more easily digested by individuals with intestinal issues.

Root Vegetable Salad

This root salad has a nice texture and color. It will go well with any traditional fall or winter dish and will make your home smell like a holiday meal.

INGREDIENTS | SERVES 4

1 rutabaga, peeled and cubed

1 turnip, peeled and cubed

6 parsnips, peeled and cubed

3 tablespoons olive oil

1 tablespoon cinnamon

3 cloves garlic, chopped

1 tablespoon ground ginger

1 teaspoon ground black pepper

1. Preheat over to 400°F.

2. Place rutabaga, turnip, and parsnips in roasting pan and drizzle with olive oil.

3. Sprinkle with cinnamon, garlic, ginger, and pepper.

4. Toss in pan to coat and roast for 40–50 minutes or until toothpick slides through vegetables easily.

PER SERVING Calories: 247 | Fat: 11 g | Protein: 4 g | Sodium: 79 mg | Fiber: 11 g | Carbohydrate: 36 g

Root Vegetables

Roots are underappreciated parts of plants. These underground vegetables are Paleo approved and recommended as they are high in vitamin A and are a nice form of carbohydrate fuel to eat, particularly post exercise.

Wasabi Mayonnaise

Traditional wasabi paste is made with real mayonnaise. This version is Paleo friendly and can be used with sushi or other types of proteins.

INGREDIENTS | SERVE 8

2 large eggs

2 tablespoons lemon juice

1 teaspoon mustard powder

2 tablespoons wasabi powder

1½ cups grapeseed oil

1. Combine eggs, lemon juice, mustard powder, and wasabi powder in a food processor and pulse until blended.

2. Drizzle grapeseed oil into egg mixture slowly and continue to pulse until completely blended.

PER SERVING Calories: 382 | Fat: 42 g | Protein: 2 g | Sodium: 16 mg | Fiber: 0 g | Carbohydrate: 1 g

Eating Raw Proteins

There has been some debate whether or not you should eat protein raw. There are certain vitamins that are diminished in the cooking process, like C, B_6, and B_9, but others, like egg protein, are more digestible.

Sesame Mayonnaise

This dressing is great on beef, turkey, or chicken burgers.

INGREDIENTS | **SERVES 8**

2 large eggs
2 tablespoons lemon juice
1 teaspoon mustard powder
2 tablespoons tahini paste
1½ cups grapeseed oil

1. Combine eggs, lemon juice, mustard powder, and tahini paste in a food processor and pulse until blended.

2. Drizzle grapeseed oil into egg mixture slowly and continue to pulse until completely blended.

PER SERVING Calories: 402 | Fat: 44 g | Protein: 2 g | Sodium: 20 mg | Fiber: 0.5 g | Carbohydrate: 1 g

Chipotle Mayonnaise

This dressing will add a nice flavor to most meat, poultry, or fish dishes.

INGREDIENTS | SERVES 8

2 large eggs

2 tablespoons lemon juice

1 teaspoon mustard powder

2 tablespoons minced chipotle peppers

1½ cups grapeseed oil

1. Place eggs, lemon juice, mustard powder, and chipotle peppers into food processor and pulse until blended.

2. Drizzle grapeseed oil into egg mixture slowly and continue to pulse until completely blended.

PER SERVING Calories: 379 | Fat: 42 g | Protein: 1.5 g | Sodium: 16 mg | Fiber: 0 g | Carbohydrate: 0 g

Serrano-Mint Sauce

This mint sauce is great with fish, poultry, and steak. Use this in place of other condiments or as a salad dressing.

INGREDIENTS | SERVES 6

1 cup tightly packed mint leaves

2 serrano chilies, chopped

4 cloves garlic, chopped

1" piece fresh ginger, peeled and chopped

¼ cup lime juice

2 tablespoons olive oil

Combine all ingredients into food processor and pulse to coarsely blend.

PER SERVING Calories: 41 │ Fat: 4.5 g │ Protein: 0 g │ Sodium: 0.5 mg │ Fiber: 0 g │ Carbohydrate: 0 g

Habanero-Basil Sauce

This sauce is very spicy and goes well with meats and poultry.

INGREDIENTS | SERVES 6

2 cups chopped basil leaves

3 habanero peppers, stemmed

2 cloves garlic

¼ cup lime juice

3 tablespoons olive oil

Combine all ingredients into food processor and pulse to coarsely blend.

PER SERVING Calories: 66 | Fat: 7 g | Protein: 0.5 g | Sodium: 1 mg | Fiber: 1 g | Carbohydrate: 1 g

Curry Salad Dressing

This dressing goes well on any salad and has a nice flavor from the curry powder.

INGREDIENTS | SERVES 1

3 tablespoons olive oil

Juice of 1 lime

1 teaspoon curry powder

½ teaspoon ground black pepper

1 teaspoon dried basil

Combine all ingredients in bowl and stir well. Serve immediately on salad.

PER SERVING Calories: 370 | Fat: 41 g | Protein: 0.5 g | Sodium: 3 mg | Fiber: 1 g | Carbohydrate: 2 g

Asian Dressing

This dressing is perfect with poultry. When you crave the taste of Chinese food, add this recipe to any plain dish to spice things up a bit.

INGREDIENTS | SERVES 4

2 tablespoons olive oil

2 tablespoons sesame oil

2 tablespoons tahini paste

½ teaspoon ground black pepper

1 teaspoon dried thyme leaves

Combine all ingredients, mix well, and serve on salad.

PER SERVING Calories: 165 | Fat: 18 g | Protein: 1.5 g | Sodium: 9 mg | Fiber: 1 g | Carbohydrate: 1.5 g

Lemon-Dill Dressing

This traditional dressing is best on fish recipes.

INGREDIENTS | **SERVES 2**

2 tablespoons olive oil

Juice of 1 lemon

1 teaspoon fresh dill

½ teaspoon ground black pepper

Combine all ingredients, mix well, and serve on salad.

PER SERVING Calories: 120 | Fat: 14 g | Protein: 0 g | Sodium: 0.5 g | Fiber: 0 g | Carbohydrate: 0 g

Oils

Many salad dressing recipes call for olive oil, but you should feel free to experiment with various oils. Each oil has a different flavor and, more important, a different fat profile. Flaxseed oil is higher in omega-3 fatty acid than others. Walnut oil has a lower omega-6 to omega-3 ratio compared with others. Uddo's oil is a nice blend of oils with various omega-3s, 6s, and 9s. These oils together have a nice flavor and have the best to offer in fat profile.

Walnut-Parsley Pesto

Walnuts add a significant blast of omega-3 fatty acids to this delicious pesto.

INGREDIENTS | SERVES 4

½ cup walnuts

8 cloves garlic

1 bunch parsley, roughly chopped

¼ cup olive oil

Freshly cracked black pepper, to taste

Pesto for All

Pesto is a generic term for anything made by pounding. Most people are familiar with traditional pesto, which is made with basil and pine nuts, but many prefer this variation with parsley and walnuts.

1. Chop the walnuts in a food processor or blender. Add the garlic and process to form a paste. Add the parsley; pulse into the walnut mixture.

2. While the blender is running, drizzle in the oil until the mixture is smooth. Add pepper to taste.

PER SERVING Calories: 229 | Fat: 23 g | Protein: 3 g | Sodium: 6 mg | Fiber: 1 g | Carbohydrate: 4 g

Red Pepper Coulis

Coulis can be made using any fruit or vegetable. To add variety, experiment with the addition of herbs and spices.

INGREDIENTS | SERVES 8

6 red peppers
1 tablespoon olive oil
Freshly cracked black pepper, to taste

1. Preheat oven to 375°F.

2. Toss the red peppers with the oil in a medium-size bowl. Place the peppers on a racked sheet pan and put in the oven for 15–20 minutes, until the skins begin to blister and the red peppers wilt.

3. Remove from oven and immediately place the red peppers in a glass or ceramic container with a top. Let sit for approximately 5 minutes, then peel off the skin from the peppers. Stem, seed, and dice the peppers.

4. Place the red peppers in a blender and purée until smooth. Season with black pepper.

PER SERVING Calories: 39 | Fat: 1.5 g | Protein: 0.5 g | Sodium: 1.5 mg | Fiber: 1.5 g | Carbohydrate: 6 g

Orange Salad

A healthful salad that makes a visual impact.

INGREDIENTS | SERVES 4

3 cups cubed butternut squash, drizzled with olive oil and roasted

2 carrots, shredded

2 cups diced papaya

2 tablespoons shredded fresh ginger

Juice of 1 lime

1 tablespoon honey, or to taste

1 tablespoon olive oil

Freshly ground black pepper

1. Combine the squash, carrots, and papaya in a large salad bowl. Set aside.

2. Stir together the ginger, lime juice, honey, olive oil, salt, and pepper until well combined. Toss the dressing with the salad ingredients and serve.

PER SERVING Calories: 160 | Fat: 4 g | Protein: 1 g | Sodium: 32 mg | Fiber: 7 g | Carbohydrate: 28 g

Mediterranean Tomato Salad

Use juicy tomatoes for this recipe, such as heirloom or beefsteak. You can substitute orange bell pepper for the yellow if needed.

INGREDIENTS | SERVES 4

2 cups tomatoes, sliced

1 cup cucumber, peeled and chopped

⅓ cup yellow bell pepper, diced

¼ cup radishes, sliced

¼ cup flat-leaf parsley, chopped

1 garlic clove, finely minced

1 tablespoon lemon juice

3 tablespoons extra-virgin olive oil

2 cups baby spinach leaves, torn

Salt and pepper, to taste

1. Toss tomatoes, cucumbers, bell pepper, radishes, and parsley together in a large salad bowl.

2. Sprinkle garlic, lemon juice, and oil over salad. Toss to coat. Salt and pepper to taste. Split spinach between four plates and top with salad. Serve immediately.

PER SERVING Calories: 131 | Fat: 10 g | Protein: 2.5 g | Sodium: 71 mg | Fiber: 2.5 g | Carbohydrate: 7 g

Kale and Sea Vegetables with Orange Sesame Dressing

This salad is a great appetizer for an Asian-themed meal.

INGREDIENTS | SERVES 4

¼ cup wakame seaweed

½ cup sea lettuce

3 cups kale

½ teaspoon lemon juice

¼ cup fresh squeezed orange juice

6 tablespoons sesame seeds (additional for garnish)

1 tablespoon kelp powder

Sea Vegetables

Sea vegetables are among the most nutritious and mineral-rich foods on earth. Ocean water contains all the mineral elements known to man. For example, both kelp and dulse are excellent sources of iodine, which is an essential nutrient missing in most diets. Sea vegetables are dried and should be soaked in water to reconstitute before eating.

1. Soak the wakame and sea lettuce in water for 30 minutes. Rinse and discard the soak water.

2. Remove the stems from the kale. Roll up the kale leaves and chop into small pieces.

3. Sprinkle lemon juice onto the kale and massage it by hand to create a wilting effect.

4. Place the orange juice, sesame seeds, and kelp powder into a blender and blend until smooth.

5. Toss the dressing with the kale and sea vegetables in a large bowl until well covered. Sprinkle about 1 teaspoon sesame seeds on top.

PER SERVING Calories: 90 | Fat: 5 g | Protein: 4 g | Sodium: 64 mg | Fiber: 3 g | Carbohydrate: 9 g

Spring Greens with Berries

The acid in the lime juice breaks down the fat in the olive oil to make a flavorful dressing.

INGREDIENTS | SERVES 2

1 jalapeño pepper
4 tablespoons lime juice
4 tablespoons olive oil
¼ teaspoon cumin, ground
4 cups mixed baby greens
2 cups fresh blackberries or raspberries
¼ cup red onion, thinly sliced

1. Slice the jalapeño pepper and remove the seeds and stem. Mince the pepper flesh.

2. Place the lime juice, olive oil, cumin, and 2 teaspoons of the minced jalapeño pepper in a blender and blend together until smooth.

3. Toss the dressing with the greens, berries, and onions and serve as a side salad.

PER SERVING Calories: 363 | Fat: 28 g | Protein: 5.5 g | Sodium: 242 mg | Fiber: 9.5 g | Carbohydrate: 21 g

Minty Blueberry Melon Salad

Seedless watermelons can sometimes have small white seeds scattered among the flesh. Use a fork to remove any noticeable seeds from the cubed watermelon before making the salad.

INGREDIENTS | SERVES 4

1½ cups cantaloupe, 1" cubes
1 cup seedless watermelon, 1" cubes
1 cup green grapes, halved
¾ cup blueberries
1 tablespoon mint leaves, minced
1 teaspoon flat-leaf parsley, minced

1. Gently toss the cantaloupe, watermelon, blueberries, and grapes together in a large salad bowl.

2. Add mint and parsley to salad. Toss to mix. Serve immediately or chill in fridge for up to 2 hours.

PER SERVING Calories: 65 | Fat: 0.5 g | Protein: 1.5 g | Sodium: 12 mg | Fiber: 1.5 g | Carbohydrate: 16 g

American Fruit Salad

This classic fruit salad is the perfect accompaniment for breakfast or lunch.

INGREDIENTS | SERVES 4

½ cup cantaloupe, cubed
½ cup honeydew melon, cubed
½ cup watermelon, cubed
½ cup red grapes
½ cup strawberries, quartered

1. Toss all the fruits together gently in a large bowl.

2. Chill fruit salad before serving.

3. Serve the salad family-style or divide it among four small plates.

PER SERVING Calories: 38 | Fat: 0 g | Protein: 1 g | Sodium: 8 mg | Fiber: 1 g | Carbohydrate: 9.5 g

Grape Types

Grapes are broken into two major categories: wine grapes and table grapes. Wine grapes are red and green grapes with high sugar content for wine purposes. Table grapes are red and green grapes with a lighter and slightly less sweet flavor than wine grapes, making them popular for culinary purposes.

Sweet and Fruity Salad

Always rinse fresh produce under cool water. This will help remove things you don't want to eat such as pesticides, fertilizers, and bacteria.

INGREDIENTS | SERVES 1

2 cups shredded romaine lettuce

4 cherry tomatoes

½ cup Gala apple, sliced

2 tablespoons golden raisins

2 tablespoons mandarin oranges, diced

Combine all ingredients in a bowl and enjoy.

PER SERVING Calories: 135 | Fat: 1 g | Protein: 3 g | Sodium: 18 mg | Fiber: 5 g | Carbohydrate: 33 g

Rainbow Fruit Salad

You can't go wrong with this salad—it's juicy, fresh, naturally low in fat and sodium, and cholesterol free. Enjoy it as a salad or as a dessert.

INGREDIENTS | SERVES 12

1 large mango, peeled and diced

2 cups fresh blueberries

1 cup bananas, sliced

2 cups fresh strawberries, halved

2 cups seedless grapes

1 cup nectarines, unpeeled, sliced

½ cup kiwi fruit, peeled, sliced

⅓ cup fresh squeezed orange juice

2 tablespoons lemon juice

1½ tablespoons honey

¼ teaspoon ginger, ground

⅛ teaspoon nutmeg, ground

1. Gently toss mango, blueberries, bananas, strawberries, grapes, nectarines, and kiwi together in a large mixing bowl.

2. Stir orange juice, lemon juice, honey, ginger, and nutmeg together in a small bowl and mix well.

3. Chill fruit until needed, up to 3 hours. Just before serving, pour honey-orange sauce over fruit and toss gently to coat.

PER SERVING Calories: 83 | Fat: 0.5 g | Protein: 1.5 g | Sodium: 2 mg | Fiber: 3 g | Carbohydrate: 21 g

Arugula and Fennel Salad with Pomegranate

Pomegranates pack a high dose of beneficial health-promoting antioxidants. They are in peak season October through January and can be substituted with dried cranberries if unavailable at your local market.

INGREDIENTS | SERVES 4

2 large navel oranges
1 pomegranate
4 cups arugula
1 cup fennel, thinly sliced
4 tablespoons olive oil
Pepper, to taste

Fennel Facts

Fennel, a crunchy and slightly sweet vegetable, is a popular Mediterranean ingredient. Fennel has a white or greenish-white bulb and long stalks with feathery green leaves stemming from the top. Fennel is closely related to cilantro, dill, carrots, and parsley.

1. Cut the tops and bottoms off of the oranges and then cut the remaining peel away from the oranges. Slice each orange into 10–12 small pieces.

2. Remove seeds from the pomegranate.

3. Place arugula, orange pieces, pomegranate seeds, and fennel slices into a large bowl.

4. Coat the salad with olive oil and season with pepper as desired.

PER SERVING Calories: 224 | Fat: 15 g | Protein: 3 g | Sodium: 22 mg | Fiber: 6 g | Carbohydrates: 24 g

Salmon-Spinach Salad

This salad makes perfect use of leftover salmon! Salmon will only remain good in the fridge for 2 days, so make sure you find a good use for it quickly!

INGREDIENTS | **SERVES 1**

1 (5-ounce) salmon fillet, cooked

1 cup spinach leaves

½ cup red grapes

¼ cup shredded carrots

1 tablespoon sliced almonds

1 tablespoon fresh raspberries

Combine ingredients in a bowl and enjoy.

PER SERVING Calories | Fat: 9 g | Protein: 24 g | Sodium: 94 mg | Fiber: 3 g | Carbohydrate: 20 g

Pineapple Onion Salad

This sweet and tangy recipe does not keep well, so make sure to throw it together right before eating. If you prefer a little more zing, add another tablespoon of lime juice and a sprinkle of cayenne pepper.

INGREDIENTS | SERVES 4

1 cup fresh pineapple, cubed
½ cup red onion, chopped
3 cups mixed baby greens
1 tablespoon lime juice

1. Place pineapple chunks in a large salad bowl. Mix onions and baby greens into the pineapple.

2. Sprinkle lightly with lime juice. Toss to coat and serve immediately.

PER SERVING Calories: 28 | Fat: 0 g | Protein: 0 g | Sodium: 1 mg | Fiber: 1 g | Carbohydrate: 5.5 g

Turkey and Cranberry Salad on Butternut Squash

This recipe offers a new twist on an American classic with a Mediterranean flair.

INGREDIENTS | SERVES 6

1 butternut squash
⅛ teaspoon nutmeg, ground
12 ounces turkey (fresh roasted)
¾ cup fresh cranberries
2 tablespoons extra-virgin olive oil
3 tablespoons fresh squeezed orange juice
Pepper, to taste

1. Preheat oven to 350°F.

2. Peel the butternut squash and cut it in half lengthwise. Remove and rinse the seeds, and place the seeds on a baking sheet; toast for approximately 5–10 minutes, until golden.

3. Thinly slice the butternut squash lengthwise into ¾ to 1" thick pieces. Brush another baking sheet with oil and lay out the squash slices; sprinkle with nutmeg. Roast the squash for approximately 20–30 minutes, until fork tender.

4. Let cool, then place the squash on plates. Arrange the turkey on top and sprinkle cranberries over the turkey. Drizzle with orange juice and oil. Season with pepper to taste.

PER SERVING Calories: 161 | Fat: 5 g | Protein: 10 g | Sodium: 334 mg | Fiber: 3.5 g | Carbohydrate: 22 g

Shaved Fennel Salad with Orange Sections and Toasted Hazelnuts

Tangelos, mandarin, or any easily sectioned citrus will work wonderfully with this recipe.

INGREDIENTS | **SERVES 6**

3 bulbs fennel

6 oranges, large

1 teaspoon hazelnuts, finely chopped

⅓ cup fresh orange juice

2 tablespoons extra-virgin olive oil

1 tablespoon fresh orange zest

1. Finely slice the fennel bulbs. Remove the peel and pith from the oranges. With a small paring knife, remove each section of the oranges and slice away membrane.

2. Form a mound of shaved fennel on each serving plate and arrange the oranges on top. Sprinkle with nuts, then drizzle with the orange juice and oil. Finish with a sprinkle of zest.

PER SERVING Calories: 172 | Fat: 5 g | Protein: 3 g | Sodium: 61 mg | Fiber: 7 g | Carbohydrate: 32 g

Blood Orange Salad with Shrimp and Baby Spinach

For an elegant supper or luncheon salad, this is a crowd pleaser. The deep red flesh of the blood oranges contrasted with the saturated green of spinach and the bright pink shrimp make for a dramatic presentation!

INGREDIENTS | **SERVES 4**

6 cups baby spinach

2 blood oranges

1¼ pounds shrimp, cleaned, cooked, and chilled

2 tablespoons fresh lemon juice

¼ cup extra-virgin olive oil

¼ teaspoon dry mustard

¼ cup stemmed, loosely packed parsley

Fresh Spinach—Not Lettuce

When you can, substitute fresh baby spinach for less nutritious iceberg lettuce. White or pale green lettuce can be used as accents but have less nutritional substance than such greens as spinach, escarole, and watercress.

1. Place the spinach on individual serving plates.

2. Peel the oranges. Slice them crossways, about ¼" thick, picking out any seeds. Arrange on top of the spinach. Arrange the shrimp around the oranges.

3. Place the rest of the ingredients in the blender and purée until the dressing is a bright green. Pour over the salads. Serve chilled.

PER SERVING Calories: 286 | Fat: 16 g | Protein: 24 g | Sodium: 194 mg | Fiber: 3 g | Carbohydrate: 14 g

Fire-Kissed Cantaloupe Salad

Garnish this light and spicy salad with fresh cilantro or a slice of mango. Serve it as a side to any filling meat dish.

INGREDIENTS | SERVES 4

2 tablespoons mango juice

1 tablespoon walnut oil

⅛ teaspoon chili powder

⅛ teaspoon sweet Hungarian paprika

⅛ teaspoon red pepper, ground

3 cups cantaloupe, cubed

½ cup red onion, diced

1. Whisk mango juice, oil, chili powder, paprika, and red pepper together in a small bowl. Whisk until salt dissolves and oil is emulsified.

2. Add cantaloupe and red onion to a large mixing bowl. Pour dressing over salad. Toss well to mix and coat. Cover salad and let chill in refrigerator for 15 minutes. Remove bowl from refrigerator, toss salad gently to mix, and serve.

PER SERVING Calories: 291 | Fat: 27 g | Protein: 1.5 g | Sodium: 41 mg | Fiber: 1.5 g | Carbohydrate: 11 g

Nuts and Trail Mixes

Blueberry Trail Mix

This trail mix recipe is the perfect blend of fruit and nuts to cure any hunger pangs. Seeds have a better omega-6 to omega-3 profile to get maximum anti-inflammatory action. The antioxidants fight free radicals.

INGREDIENTS | SERVES 2

¼ cup fresh or dried blueberries

¼ cup pumpkin seeds

1 ounce almonds

Dash cinnamon

Combine all ingredients into quart-size plastic baggie, shake, and enjoy.

PER SERVING Calories: 241 | Fat: 19 g | Protein: 13 g | Sodium: 5.5 mg | Fiber: 3 g | Carbohydrate: 9 g

Antioxidants

Antioxidants are important for attacking free radicals in your body. You really can't eat enough foods containing these important compounds. Feel free to mix up the type of berry you add to this mix. Dehydrated varieties are currently available in produce sections. These go particularly well with trail mix as spoilage factor is removed from the equation.

Nutty Chocolate Trail Mix

When you're craving something sweet, throw this quick trail mix together for a healthy alternative to a chocolate bar.

INGREDIENTS | **SERVES 4**

8 ounces organic turkey jerky
½ cup macadamia nuts
½ cup walnuts
½ cup unsweetened coconut flakes
½ cup cacao nibs

1. Cut up turkey jerky into bite-sized pieces and place in medium bowl.

2. Add remaining ingredients to bowl, mix, and serve.

PER SERVING Calories: 549 | Fat: 34 g | Protein: 23 g | Sodium: 1,058 mg | Fiber: 5 g | Carbohydrate: 20 g

Super Food Trail Mix

This mix is packed with lots of super foods for maximum health benefits in every bite.

INGREDIENTS | **SERVES 2**

½ cup pistachio nuts

½ cup cacao nibs

½ cup dried goji berries

½ cup dried mulberries

8 ounces organic buffalo jerky, cut into bite-sized pieces

Combine all ingredients, mix, and serve.

PER SERVING Calories: 540 | Fat: 37 g | Protein: 46 g | Sodium: 1,018 mg | Fiber: 7 g | Carbohydrate: 36 g

Sweet-Spicy Nut Mix

When you can't decide if you have a sweet or spicy craving, this nut mix will satisfy both.

INGREDIENTS | SERVES 10

2 teaspoons ground ginger

2 teaspoons ground cinnamon

2 teaspoons ground cumin

¼ teaspoon ground cloves

1 teaspoon chili powder

2 large egg whites

1 medium-sized mango, peeled and chopped

2 cups raw almonds

1 cup walnuts

1 cup pecans

1 cup cashews

Omega-6 and Omega-3 in Nuts

It is a good idea to add a variety of nuts to your diet. The fatty acid profile is different per nut so the variety will help you get the best overall ratios. Additionally, mixing up nuts with seeds is the best idea as seeds' ratio of omega-6 to omega-3 is much lower than nuts.

1. Preheat oven to 225°F and line 2 cookie sheets with parchment paper.

2. In a small bowl, mix together ginger, cinnamon, cumin, cloves, and chili powder.

3. In a large bowl, whisk egg whites until foamy. Whisk in spice mixture.

4. Pulse mango in a food processor until chunky. Add to egg mixture.

5. Add remaining ingredients and toss to coat the nuts.

6. Divide nut mixture evenly between the two baking sheets.

7. Bake 1½ hours, or until nuts are dry and toasted. Stir every 20 minutes.

PER SERVING Calories: 352 | Fat: 31 g | Protein: 10 g | Sodium: 15 mg | Fiber: 5 g | Carbohydrate: 14 g

Traditional Trail Mix

*This trail mix has less sugar than conventional non-Paleolithic diet trail mixes.
For a different flavor, add a different nut or dehydrated fruit.*

INGREDIENTS | SERVES 4

1 cup raw or roasted almonds

1 cup pumpkin seeds

½ cup sunflower seeds

1 cup dehydrated strawberries

½ cup goji berries

Combine all ingredients in an airtight container and store in a cool, dry place.

PER SERVING Calories: 548 | Fat: 44 g | Protein: 27 g | Sodium: 14 mg | Fiber: 8 g | Carbohydrate: 22 g

Arugula-Walnut Salad

Arugula is a nice change from the usual lettuce- or spinach-leaf salads. It has a slightly bitter taste that goes well with the warm dressing in this recipe.

INGREDIENTS | SERVES 1

4 ounces ground turkey

¾ cup walnut pieces

1 tablespoon minced shallots

1 tablespoon puréed passion fruit or mango

3 tablespoons lemon juice

½ cup walnut oil

½ teaspoon ground black pepper

8 cups baby arugula

1. Heat a small skillet over medium-high heat. Brown the ground turkey, approximately 8 minutes. Drain and set aside.

2. In a separate skillet, toast the walnuts.

3. Mix the shallots, fruit purée, and lemon juice in a medium bowl.

4. Whisk in walnut oil slowly and add black pepper.

5. Stir in walnuts.

6. Pour walnut mixture over baby arugula and top with ground turkey.

PER SERVING Calories: 447 | Fat: 42 g | Protein: 12 g | Sodium: 12 mg | Fiber: 3 g | Carbohydrate: 12 g

Asparagus and Cashew Nuts

Serve this dish as an accompaniment to fish, chicken, turkey, or beef.

INGREDIENTS | **SERVES 2**

2 tablespoons olive oil

2 tablespoons sesame oil

1 teaspoon minced fresh gingerroot

1 bunch asparagus, ends trimmed and cut into 2" pieces

1 teaspoon red pepper flakes

½ cup chopped cashews

Sesame Oil

Sesame oil is great for stir-frying. It has a high heat capacity and a relatively low smoke value so it cooks well under higher heat conditions. Additionally, sesame oil adds a nice Asian flavor to meals cooked with the oil.

1. Heat olive oil and sesame oil in a wok or sauté pan over low to medium heat.

2. Add ginger and stir-fry until slightly brown, about 5 minutes.

3. Add asparagus and red pepper flakes, and stir-fry for 3 minutes

4. Add cashews.

5. Cook until asparagus is tender, stirring frequently, about 5 minutes.

PER SERVING Calories: 466 | Fat: 43 g | Protein: 8 g | Sodium: 9 mg | Fiber: 4 g | Carbohydrate: 17 g

Pecan-Crusted Chicken

This gourmet-style meal is simple to put together, but big on flavor.
The quick fry helps to lock in moisture of the chicken.

INGREDIENTS | **SERVES 4**

4 skinless, boneless chicken breast halves

2 large eggs

¼ cup almond milk

½ cup almond meal

1½ tablespoons ground cinnamon

1 cup finely chopped pecans

½ teaspoon ground black pepper

2 tablespoons olive oil

Nut Milks

Nut milks can be used in conventional recipes calling for dairy, cream, or milk. Experiment with different kinds of nut milk. Coconut milk is thicker and adds a nice flavor. Almond milk is rather plain, mimicking the taste of regular milk quite nicely. Hazelnut milk has a great flavor and may be best used in coffee.

1. Pound chicken breasts to ½" thickness

2. In a shallow dish, beat the eggs with the almond milk.

3. In a second shallow dish, mix together almond meal, cinnamon, pecans, and pepper.

4. Dip the chicken in the egg mix, and press in the pecan mix.

5. Heat olive oil in a skillet over medium-high heat. Fry chicken breasts in hot olive oil until golden, about 5 minutes per side.

PER SERVING Calories: 500 | Fat: 21 g | Protein: 42 g | Sodium: 45 mg | Fiber: 4 g | Carbohydrate: 17 g

Pistachio-Pumpkin Trail Mix

This trail mix is sure to satisfy an active family on the go. Feel free to mix up the types of nuts or fruits you add in to make it your own personal trail mix.

INGREDIENTS | SERVES 4

½ cup pistachio nuts
½ cup pumpkin seeds
½ cup sunflower seeds
½ cup coconut flakes
1 cup dried mulberries

Combine all ingredients and serve.

PER SERVING Calories: 389 | Fat: 31 g | Protein: 17 g | Sodium: 12 mg | Fiber: 6 g | Carbohydrate: 17 g

Pecan-Crusted Catfish

Catfish and tilapia rank among the most popular fish in the United States today. They are relatively inexpensive and have a nice flavor. You can use either fish in this recipe.

INGREDIENTS | SERVES 4

½ cup almond meal
½ cup pecans, finely chopped
¼ teaspoon ground black pepper
1½ pounds catfish
2 tablespoons coconut oil

1. In a shallow dish, mix almond meal, pecans, and pepper.

2. Dredge the catfish in the pecan mixture; coating well.

3. Add coconut oil to sauté pan over medium-high heat.

4. Place catfish in pan and fry 3–5 minutes on each side.

PER SERVING Calories: 331 | Fat: 21 g | Protein: 23 g | Sodium: 60 mg | Fiber: 2.5 g | Carbohydrate: 14 g

CHAPTER 18

Desserts and Sweets

Banana Bread

This banana bread is a nice dessert or breakfast treat. You can intensify the flavor by adding more ripe bananas.

INGREDIENTS | SERVES 8

1¼ cups almond meal

2 teaspoons baking powder

¼ teaspoon baking soda

½ cup fruit purée of your choice

¼ teaspoon cinnamon

½ teaspoon vanilla extract

2 large eggs

3 large ripe bananas, mashed

¼ cup flaxseed flour

½ cup chopped walnuts

½ cup unsweetened coconut flakes

Bananas

Bananas are a great fruit, but they do raise your blood sugar significantly. In order to maximize the influx of sugar, these are always best when eaten after a workout or race.

1. Preheat oven to 350°F. Spray a loaf pan with cooking spray.

2. In a large bowl, combine almond meal, baking powder, baking soda, fruit purée, cinnamon, and vanilla.

3. Add eggs, banana, and flaxseed flour. Mix well.

4. Add walnuts and coconut flakes and fold them into the batter.

5. Bake for 45 minutes.

6. Cool in pan for 5 minutes, then transfer to wire rack to cool completely.

PER SERVING Calories: 254 | Fat: 10 g | Protein: 6 g | Sodium: 65 mg | Fiber: 6 g | Carbohydrate: 39 g

Delicious Pumpkin Pudding

This pumpkin pudding is a great dessert for the holidays.

INGREDIENTS | SERVES 8

2 large eggs
1 teaspoon cinnamon
½ teaspoon nutmeg
½ teaspoon cloves
½ teaspoon ginger
1 (15-ounce) can organic pumpkin
1 (13.5-ounce) can coconut milk
½ cup crushed pecans

Pumpkin: A Starchy Carbohydrate

Pumpkin is a fruit, but should be considered a complex carbohydrate. It will raise your insulin levels when eaten. These are always best eaten after exercise or when the sugar will be used to replenish glycogen storage. For that reason, eating high-glycemic-load items at bedtime is not recommended.

1. Preheat oven to 375°F. Grease an 8" × 8" square baking pan.

2. Whisk eggs in a medium bowl. Add spices and whisk again.

3. Add pumpkin and coconut milk and mix thoroughly.

4. Pour batter into prepared pan, top with pecans, and bake for 45 minutes.

PER SERVING Calories: 200 | Fat: 18 g | Protein: 4 g | Sodium: 26 mg | Fiber: 3 g | Carbohydrate: 8.5 g

Heavenly Cookie Bars

*These cookie bars are amazing! Keep in mind that these bars contain dried fruit,
which is not for those following a strict Paleolithic diet regime.*

INGREDIENTS | **SERVES 48**

2 cups raw honey

4 cups almond flour

½ teaspoon nutmeg

½ teaspoon ginger

½ cup dried dates, chopped

2 cups ground walnuts

½ cup raisins

1. Preheat oven to 350°F.

2. Line 2 cookie sheets with parchment paper.

3. Warm honey in a saucepan over low heat and let cool slightly.

4. Sift together flour and spices in a medium bowl.

5. Add honey to flour mixture and stir until well blended.

6. Stir in dates, walnuts, and raisins.

7. Roll dough to ¼" thick and cut into squares.

8. Place squares on prepared cookie sheets and bake for 10 minutes.

PER SERVING Calories: 121 | Fat: 3.5 g | Protein: 2.5 g |
Sodium: 1.5 g | Fiber: 2 g | Carbohydrate: 23 g

Whoopie Pies

These sweet treats are exquisite. You will be shocked at how amazing they really are. But beware, these pies have quite a few calories even though they are technically Paleo approved.

INGREDIENTS | SERVES 12

2 cups almond flour
½ cup coconut flour
½ teaspoon baking soda
1 tablespoon cinnamon
1 teaspoon dried ginger
½ teaspoon allspice
½ teaspoon nutmeg
¼ teaspoon cloves
1 cup raw honey
2 large eggs
1 tablespoon vanilla extract
¼ cup hazelnut flour

Baking Soda

Strict Paleo followers would debate that baking soda is not allowed in the Paleo-lithic lifestyle. If you are choosing to be a less-strict follower, then baking soda is allowed, but realize that this is not follow-ing the true Paleolithic lifestlye.

1. Preheat the oven to 350°F. Cover two cookie sheets with parchment paper.

2. Mix almond flour, coconut flour, baking soda, cinnamon, ginger, allspice, nutmeg, and cloves in a large bowl.

3. Add honey, eggs, and vanilla to flour mixture.

4. Add hazelnut flour and mix to form a stiff dough.

5. Place ¼-cup scoops of dough onto cookie sheets, spacing cookies 2" apart.

6. Bake for 15 minutes. Cool on wire rack.

7. If desired, sandwich two cookies with Creamy Vanilla Frosting (see this chapter).

PER SERVING Calories: 188 | Fat: 1.5 g | Protein: 4.5 g | Sodium: 65 mg | Fiber: 3 g | Carbohydrate: 43 g

Creamy Vanilla Frosting

This frosting can be used for Whoopie Pies, but also can be used to frost any dessert.

INGREDIENTS | SERVES 12

4 tablespoons coconut butter

2 tablespoons raw honey

½ cup cacao nibs

½ teaspoon vanilla extract

½ teaspoon cinnamon

Blend all ingredients in a medium bowl and whisk thoroughly.

PER SERVING Calories: 73 | Fat: 4 g | Protein: 1 g | Sodium: 3.8 mg | Fiber: 1 g | Carbohydrate: 9 g

Almond Butter Cookies

Almond cookies are a great snack. They provide you with essential fatty acids omega-6 and omega-3. Almonds are also a source of vitamin E.

INGREDIENTS | SERVES 12

1 cup almond butter

1 large egg white

2 tablespoons unsweetened applesauce

2 tablespoons unsweetened coconut flakes

1 tablespoon cacao powder

1. Preheat oven to 375°F.

2. Beat all ingredients together to form a thick batter.

3. Place tablespoon-sized scoops of dough onto an ungreased cookie sheet. Bake 10–12 minutes or until lightly brown on top.

PER SERVING Calories: 151 | Fat: 14 g | Protein: 3.8 g | Sodium: 8.6 mg | Fiber: 1.5 g | Carbohydrate: 5.5 g

Chocolate Chip Cookies

These are not quite Toll House cookies, but they are a good Paleolithic diet alternative to high-sugar and high-fat cookies.

INGREDIENTS | **SERVES 12**

1 cup sunflower butter
1 cup honey
1 large egg
2 teaspoons baking soda
1⅓ cups almond meal
¾ cup cacao nibs

1. Preheat oven to 350°F.

2. Line a baking sheet with parchment paper.

3. In a mixer, combine sunflower butter and honey until well mixed.

4. Add egg and baking soda and mix for 2 minutes.

5. Add almond meal and mix, then add cacao nibs.

6. Spoon the dough onto baking sheet and bake for 10–15 minutes until lightly browned.

7. Remove to wire rack and cool completely.

PER SERVING Calories: 286 | Fat: 14 g | Protein: 4 g | Sodium: 12 mg | Fiber: 2 g | Carbohydrate: 39 g

Chocolate Coconut Milk Balls

These coconut milk balls are not as creamy as ice cream, but are a nice alternative. You can change the flavor by changing the fruit purée that you add into the recipe.

INGREDIENTS | SERVES 10

12 tablespoons raw cacao powder

6 tablespoons fresh fruit purée of your choice

6 tablespoons coconut oil

6 tablespoons coconut milk

3 tablespoons unsweetened shredded coconut

2 tablespoons cacao nibs

1 ripe banana

1. Combine all ingredients in food processor and pulse until very smooth.

2. Add water if the consistency is not fluid.

3. Pour into ice cube trays or molds and freeze.

PER SERVING Calories: 149 | Fat: 13 g | Protein: 2 g | Sodium: 4 mg | Fiber: 3.5 g | Carbohydrate: 11 g

Coconut

Coconut has many great properties. This recipe uses all the edible parts of the coconut—the meat, oil, and milk. You will receive high fiber, vitamin, and mineral content as well as skin benefits from consumption of coconut. It is a Paleolithic dieter's best friend.

Baked Bananas

This healthy dessert is sure to be a favorite of yours. Make in bulk and use to spread on Paleo pancakes or Paleo banana bread.

INGREDIENTS | SERVES 4

4 small bananas, peeled
½ teaspoon grated orange rind
½ tablespoon fruit purée
1 tablespoon lemon juice
⅛ teaspoon cinnamon
⅛ teaspoon nutmeg
1 tablespoon melted coconut oil
1 tablespoon cacao nibs

1. Preheat oven to 350°F.

2. Cut each banana lengthwise and across into 8 pieces.

3. Arrange banana slices in a small baking pan.

4. Sprinkle evenly with orange rind, fruit purée, lemon juice, cinnamon, nutmeg, and coconut oil.

5. Bake uncovered 35–40 minutes, basting after 15 minutes with liquid in dish.

6. Sprinkle with cacao nibs before serving.

PER SERVING Calories: 200 | Fat: 5 g | Protein: 1.5 g | Sodium: 1.5 mg | Fiber: 5 g | Carbohydrate: 41 g

Chocolate Almond Sliver Cookies

These cookies are a nice treat without the guilt.

INGREDIENTS | SERVES 12

5 large egg whites
3 cups slivered almonds
½ cup cacao nibs
¼ cup raw honey

Nut Alternatives

Of all the nuts, almonds have the worst omega-6 to omega-3 ratio. Feel free to switch it up in recipes where nuts are included. The above recipe would work for pecans, hazelnuts, walnuts, or seeds such as sunflower or pumpkin. The great thing about these recipes is that you can alter them to fit your needs and tastes.

1. Preheat oven to 350°F. Spray cookie sheet with cooking spray.

2. Whisk egg whites for 30 seconds.

3. Add almonds, cacao nibs, and honey to egg whites and mix well.

4. Form 1" balls and place on coated cookie sheet.

5. Bake until lightly brown on top, approximately 10 minutes.

PER SERVING Calories: 197 | Fat: 14 g | Protein: 7 g | Sodium: 27 mg | Fiber: 3 g | Carbohydrate: 15 g

Paleo "Yes" Foods

In order to ensure your success on the Paleolithic diet, you need to stock your pantry with fresh, organic produce and grass-fed and barn-roaming meats. This list contains both the basics and the obscure. Feel free to experiment with items you would not normally choose. That will spice things up and keep you interested in the diet.

Protein

alligator

bass

bear

beef, lean and trimmed

bison

bluefish

caribou

chicken breast

chuck steak

clams

cod

crab

crayfish

egg whites

eggs

flank steak

game hen breasts

goat

grouper

haddock

halibut

hamburger, extra lean

herring

liver (beef, lamb, goat, or chicken)

lobster

London broil

mackerel

marrow (beef, lamb, or goat)

mussels

orange roughy

ostrich

oysters

pheasant

pork chops

pork loin

pork, lean
quail
rabbit
rattlesnake
red snapper
salmon, wild-caught
scallops
scrod
shrimp
tilapia
tongue (beef, lamb, or goat)
trout
tuna, canned, unsalted
tuna, fresh
turkey breast
veal, lean
venison

Leafy Vegetables

arugula
beet greens
bitterleaf
bok choy
broccoli rabe
Brussels sprouts
cabbage
celery
chard
chicory
Chinese cabbage
collard greens
dandelion
endive
fiddlehead
kale

lettuce
radicchio
spinach
Swiss chard
turnip
watercress
yarrow

Fruiting Vegetables

avocado
bell pepper
cucumber
eggplant
squash
sweet pepper
tomatillo
tomato
zucchini

Flowers and Flower Buds

artichoke
broccoli
cauliflower

Bulb and Stem Vegetables

asparagus
celery
Florence fennel
garlic
kohlrabi
leek
onion

Sea Vegetables and Herbs of All Types

Fruits

apple
apricot
banana
blackberries
blueberries
cantaloupe
cherries
coconut
cranberries (not dried)
figs
grapefruit
grapes
guava
honeydew melon
kiwi
lemon
lime
mandarin orange
mango
nectarine
orange
papaya
passion fruit
peaches
pears
persimmon
pineapple
plums
pomegranate
raspberries
rhubarb

star fruit
strawberries
tangerine
watermelon
All other fruits are acceptable

Fats, Nuts, Seeds, Oils, and Fatty Proteins

almond butter
almonds
avocado
brazil nuts
canola oil
cashew
cashew butter
chestnuts
coconut oil
flaxseed oil
hazelnuts/filberts
macadamia butter
macadamia nuts
olive oil
pecans
pine nuts
pistachios
pumpkin seeds
safflower oil
sesame seeds
sunflower butter, unsweetened
sunflower seeds
Uddo's oil
walnut oil
walnuts

APPENDIX B

Paleo "No" Foods

Legume Vegetables

American groundnut
azuki beans
black-eyed peas
chickpeas (garbanzo bean)
common beans
fava beans
green beans
guar
Indian peas
kidney beans
lentils
lima beans
mung beans
navy beans
okra
peanut
peanut butter
peas
pigeon peas
pinto beans
red beans
ricebeans
snow peas
soybean and soy products
string beans
sugar snap peas
white beans

Dairy Foods

all processed foods made with any dairy products
butter
cheese
cream
dairy spreads
frozen yogurt
ice cream
ice milk
low-fat milk
nonfat dairy creamer
powdered milk
skim milk
whole milk
yogurt

Cereal Grains

barley
corn
millet
oats
rice
rye
sorghum
wheat
wild rice

Cereal Grain-Like Seeds

amaranth
buckwheat
quinoa

Starchy Vegetables

starchy tubers

cassava root

manioc

potatoes and all potato products

sweet potatoes or yams (unless after workout to replenish gylcogen)

tapioca pudding

Salt-Containing Foods, Fatty Meats, and Sugar

almost all commercial salad dressings and condiments

bacon

beef ribs

candy

canned salted meat or fish

chicken and turkey legs, thighs, and wings

chicken and turkey skin

deli meats

fatty ground beef

fatty pork cuts

frankfurters

ham

ketchup

lamb roast

olives

pickled foods

pork rinds

processed meats

salami

salted nuts

salted spices

sausages

smoked, dried, and salted fish and meat

soft drinks and fruit juice

sugar

Paleo Substitutions

Paleo Substitutions	
cow's milk	coconut, almond, macadamia, or hazelnut milk
bacon	uncured bacon and meats
deli meat	fresh cut chicken or turkey breast, thinly sliced
salad dressing	oil and lemon or lime juice
vinegar	lemon or lime juice
starch	spaghetti squash, butternut squash, acorn squash
sugar	raw honey
soda	fruit-infused water, iced tea
salt	lemon juice, spices, fresh herbs
butter	nut oils, coconut butter
peanut butter	all other nut and seed butters
cookies	fresh fruit
chocolate	cacao
commercially prepared meat	grass-fed, barn-roaming meat
farm raised fish	wild-caught fish
baked desserts	baked fruit

Standard U.S./Metric Measurement Conversions

VOLUME CONVERSIONS	
U.S. Volume Measure	**Metric Equivalent**
⅛ teaspoon	0.5 milliliters
¼ teaspoon	1 milliliters
½ teaspoon	2 milliliters
1 teaspoon	5 milliliters
½ tablespoon	7 milliliters
1 tablespoon (3 teaspoons)	15 milliliters
2 tablespoons (1 fluid ounce)	30 milliliters
¼ cup (4 tablespoons)	60 milliliters
⅓ cup	90 milliliters
½ cup (4 fluid ounces)	125 milliliters
⅔ cup	160 milliliters
¾ cup (6 fluid ounces)	180 milliliters
1 cup (16 tablespoons)	250 milliliters
1 pint (2 cups)	500 milliliters
1 quart (4 cups)	1 liter (about)

WEIGHT CONVERSIONS	
U.S. Weight Measure	**Metric Equivalent**
½ ounce	15 grams
1 ounce	30 grams
2 ounces	60 grams
3 ounces	85 grams
¼ pound (4 ounces)	115 grams
½ pound (8 ounces)	225 grams
¾ pound (12 ounces)	340 grams
1 pound (16 ounces)	454 grams

OVEN TEMPERATURE CONVERSIONS

Degrees Fahrenheit	Degrees Celsius
200 degrees F	100 degrees C
250 degrees F	120 degrees C
275 degrees F	140 degrees C
300 degrees F	150 degrees C
325 degrees F	160 degrees C
350 degrees F	180 degrees C
375 degrees F	190 degrees C
400 degrees F	200 degrees C
425 degrees F	220 degrees C
450 degrees F	230 degrees C

BAKING PAN SIZES

American	Metric
8 x 1½ inch round baking pan	20 x 4 cm cake tin
9 x 1½ inch round baking pan	23 x 3.5 cm cake tin
1 x 7 x 1½ inch baking pan	28 x 18 x 4 cm baking tin
13 x 9 x 2 inch baking pan	30 x 20 x 5 cm baking tin
2 quart rectangular baking dish	30 x 20 x 3 cm baking tin
15 x 10 x 2 inch baking pan	30 x 25 x 2 cm baking tin (Swiss roll tin)
9 inch pie plate	22 x 4 or 23 x 4 cm pie plate
7 or 8 inch springform pan	18 or 20 cm springform or loose bottom cake tin
9 x 5 x 3 inch loaf pan	23 x 13 x 7 cm or 2 lb narrow loaf or pate tin
1½ quart casserole	1.5 liter casserole
2 quart casserole	2 liter casserole

Index

Note: Page numbers in **bold** indicate recipe category lists.

We Have
EVERYTHING®
on Anything!

With more than 19 million copies sold, the Everything® series has become one of America's favorite resources for solving problems, learning new skills, and organizing lives. Our brand is not only recognizable—it's also welcomed.

The series is a hand-in-hand partner for people who are ready to tackle new subjects—like you!

For more information on the Everything® series, please visit *www.adamsmedia.com*

The Everything® list spans a wide range of subjects, with more than 500 titles covering 25 different categories:

Business	History	Reference
Careers	Home Improvement	Religion
Children's Storybooks	Everything Kids	Self-Help
Computers	Languages	Sports & Fitness
Cooking	Music	Travel
Crafts and Hobbies	New Age	Wedding
Education/Schools	Parenting	Writing
Games and Puzzles	Personal Finance	
Health	Pets	